Healing Families

A Guide to Helping Families Deal With Substance Use Disorder

Eric G. Daxon, Ph.D., CRSPS   Joanne Daxon, LCDC
Frank Janousek, CRSPS   Elizabeth Todd, LCDC

Healing Families: A Guide to Helping Families Deal with Substance Use Disorder
Eric G. Daxon, Joanne Daxon, Frank Janousek, And Elizabeth Todd

Copyright © 2024 Eric G. Daxon, Joanne Daxon, Frank Janousek, Elizabeth Todd

All Rights Reserved. Except The Appendices May Be Copied For Use In Working With Clients Or For Educational Purposes.

Imprint: Eric G. Daxon

Requests for information should be mailed to Eric G. Daxon, c/o RecoveryWerks! 790 Landa Street, New Braunfels, TX 78130
Cover and Interior Design by Caerus Kourt

Paperback ISBN: 979-8-9919481-1-1
Ebook ISBN: 979-8-9919481-3-5

Acknowledgments

First, the authors would like to thank the people who fostered our personal recoveries: our sponsors, members of our recovery groups, our recovery coaches, and our families. God has given us the gift of sobriety; these people were His tools. Second, we would like to thank Phil Sagebiel for the multiple copy edits of this book and for agreeing to provide summaries of the books in our suggested reading list. Phil is a family group member who we believe has read almost every recovery book out there—a slight exaggeration. We are especially grateful that Phil agreed to review the book when it was in its early, very rough state. Next, we would like to thank our main editor, Martha E. Lang. Her first edit of this book was, let's say, "extensive." All of her numerous edits were spot on and led to a significant and needed rewrite of the book. Her second edit was less daunting than the first but equally helpful. We would like to thank Colleen Sheehan for the stunning cover design, illustrations, book interior design, and production. Thanks, Martha and Colleen!

Table of Contents

ACKNOWLEDGMENTS		iii
TABLE OF CONTENTS		iv
FIGURES		vi
TABLES		vii
CHAPTER 1.	Introduction	1
PART I.	SUD, Codependency and the Recovery Process	5
CHAPTER 2.	Substance Use Disorder, Codependency, and Family Roles	7
CHAPTER 3.	The Family Member Recovery Process	35
PART II.	The Family Recovery Program	55
CHAPTER 4.	Integrated Alternative Peer Groups for Family Member Recovery	57
CHAPTER 5.	Integrated Alternative Peer Group Recovery Culture	61
CHAPTER 6.	Family Group Meetings	89
CHAPTER 7.	Peer Coaching/Counseling Appointments	103
CHAPTER 8.	Family Member Recovery Plan	115

PART III. Recovery Tools 133

CHAPTER 9.	Barriers to Recovery	135
CHAPTER 10.	Boundaries for Families Dealing with Substance Use Disorder	155
CHAPTER 11.	Resent, Own, Appreciate, Demand (ROAD) Tool	201
CHAPTER 12.	Living in the Moment	209
CHAPTER 13.	Strengthening a Relationship with God	217
CHAPTER 14.	Moving from Non-recovery Beliefs to Recovery Beliefs	239
CHAPTER 15.	Overcoming Guilt and Shame	257
CHAPTER 16.	Recognizing and Dealing with Grief	277
APPENDIX A:	Recovery Plan Preparation	287
APPENDIX B:	Codependency Recovery Plan	293
APPENDIX C:	Plan for Enjoyment and Fun	301
APPENDIX D:	Codependency Relapse Prevention and Relapse Recovery Plan	309
APPENDIX E:	Suggested Reading List	315
APPENDIX F:	Do You Need Boundaries in Your Life?	319
APPENDIX G:	Identify the Loved One's Unacceptable Behaviors and Family Member Enabling Behaviors	321
APPENDIX H:	Boundary-Setting Handout	323
APPENDIX I:	Example Boundaries for Minors and Adults	325

APPENDIX J:	Resent, Own, Appreciate, Demand (ROAD) Worksheet	331
APPENDIX K:	Living in the Moment	337
APPENDIX L:	AA Big Book Prayers, Your Higher Power Speaking to You	341
APPENDIX M:	Prayer and Meditation	345
APPENDIX N:	Worksheet for the Event, Emotion, Belief, Feeling, Action Process	349
APPENDIX O:	Guilt and Shame Inventory	355
REFERENCES		357

FIGURES

FIGURE 1.	Pleasure and Pain in the Four Stages of Substance Use Disorder	10
FIGURE 2.	Codependency's Progression From Normal Family Functioning to Codependency	17
FIGURE 3.	Stages of Change for Recovering from SUD and Codependency	45
FIGURE 4.	Integrated Alternative Peer Group Structure and Processes	59
FIGURE 5.	The Components of the Recovery Culture	62
FIGURE 6.	Unconditional Acceptance	72
FIGURE 7.	Core Values of a 12 Step Program	78
FIGURE 8.	Family Group Meeting Types for PDAP-style Programs	89
FIGURE 9.	Meeting Safety Guidelines	92
FIGURE 10.	General Approach to Appointments	104

FIGURE 11.	General Approach to First Appointment	107
FIGURE 12.	Process for Developing a Recovery Plan	116
FIGURE 13.	Barriers to Family Member Recovery	135
FIGURE 14.	Approach to Setting Boundaries	164
FIGURE 15.	Event, Emotion, Belief, Feeling, Action Process	240
FIGURE 16.	Notional Relationship Between Doing Right or Wrong Thing and Outcomes	261

TABLES

TABLE 1.	Spiritual Values for Each of the 12 Steps	37
TABLE 2.	Types of Love	68
TABLE 3.	The 12 Steps of AA	79
TABLE 4.	Family Member Losses when the Loved One Is Using Is in Recovery	281
TABLE 5.	Losses for the Substance User When Using and When in Recovery	283

TABLES IN THE APPENDICES

TABLE 1.	Needs Assessment	294
TABLE 2.	Action Plan Template	298
TABLE 3.	Example Action Plan	299

Healing Families

CHAPTER 1

Introduction

Substance Use Disorder (SUD) is a serious, often fatal disease that the American Psychiatric Association defines as "... a complex condition in which there is uncontrolled use of a substance despite harmful consequences. People with SUD have an intense focus on using a certain substance(s), such as alcohol, tobacco, or illicit drugs, to the point where the person's ability to function in day-to-day life becomes impaired. People keep using the substance even when they know it is causing or will cause problems. The most severe SUDs are sometimes called addictions." (American Psychiatric Association 2020)

Like all serious diseases, SUD affects the family. However, it is unique because, unlike most serious illnesses, the affected person has the compulsion to continue taking the substance that causes and worsens the disease, sometimes up to the point of dying. To family members with no understanding of SUD, the compulsion to use is both baffling and especially painful because their loved one[1] appears to be willfully harming themselves and, with malice of forethought, destroying the family. The family usually loves the person with all their heart and desperately wants to save their loved one.

Family member frustration, panic, anger, and anxiety rapidly rise when all the family's standard tools for dealing with the loved one fail and seem to

---

1 In this book, the loved one refers to the person in the family with SUD.

make the loved one's disease worse and not better. As the loved one's disease worsens, the family's deep love and desire to save heightens their desire to protect their loved one. Without help, the family member will spiral into some of the following - mental illness, bitterness, anger, divorce, isolation, debilitating regret, and SUD. The family member's downward spiral worsens the loved one's downward spiral and vice versa. This deep love and desire to save often leads to a singular focus on the loved one, which we will term codependency.[2]

All of the authors have loved ones with SUD, and all experienced this spiral. All authors received the help they needed from a Palmer Drug Abuse Program (PDAP) location. Joanne, Elizabeth, and Eric were a part of PDAP in San Antonio, TX. Frank's recovery started in the PDAP located in Hobbs, New Mexico. All authors eventually worked for PDAP or organizations that used the PDAP approach to recovery. PDAP recovery for teens and young adults centers on the alternative peer group (APG) (Palmer Drug Abuse Program - National, Inc. 1982, Palmer Drug Abuse Program 1990) The APG was specifically developed to provide teens and young adults with a group of friends who were interested in getting and staying sober. This group was an alternative to the friends the teen/young adult used substances with. Cates and Cummings termed the PDAP-style APG as an integrated APG because it integrated peer groups, 12-Step recovery, counseling, fun activities, and family support (Cates and Cummings 2003).[3]

One of the central tenets of family member recovery is that the family is not responsible

> **CODEPENDENCY**
>
> One of the central tenets of family member recovery is that the family is not responsible for their loved one's SUD. *Similarly, the loved one is not responsible for the family's turmoil.* How family members choose to respond to the loved one's SUD is the root cause of their misery.

---

2   Codependency is discussed in more detail in Chapter 2, Substance Use Disorder, Codependency, and Family Roles.

3   Chapter 4, Alternative Peer Groups for Family Member Recovery, has more information on APGs.

for their loved one's SUD. *Similarly, the loved one is not responsible for the family's misery.* How family members choose to respond to the loved one's SUD is the root cause of their misery. Family recovery occurs when each family member first confronts and addresses the enemy within - their false beliefs, resentments, and character defects. Second, they learn and apply recovery's many tools without letting fear paralyze them. Recovery cannot be done alone, but each family member is responsible for their recovery and no one else's.

There are many books written to help family members dealing with SUD. Most are self-help books written for family members to read. Several books have been written by clinicians for clinicians working with families who are coping with SUD.[4] What sets this book apart is that the authors wrote it for peer recovery coaches/counselors who want to work with family members.

The first objective of this book is to provide the recovery coach/counselor with an intellectual and emotional understanding of the impact of a loved one's SUD on a family member. Family members need a great deal of grace because they lack the knowledge, tools, and support to make the choices that will mitigate the turmoil and allow them to regain their lives.

The second objective is to provide the recovery coach with tools to help family members recover. This book is based on the integrated APG approach to family member recovery, and the tools provided align with the integrated APG approach. Specifically, this book offers the peer recovery coach with the following:

- An understanding of the integrated APG approach and how to apply it.

- A cognitive and emotional understanding of codependency and the impact this has on family members.

---

[4] Appendix E: Suggested Reading List is a listing of recommended books.

- The ability to apply the Substance Abuse and Mental Health Agency's Guiding Principles of Recovery and the stages of change to family member recovery.

- Guidance on conducting coaching appointments for family members.

- Tools to aid a family member in their recovery and to overcome their barriers to recovery.

This tool chest has three parts. Part I, SUD, Codependency and the Recovery Process, discusses the basics of SUD and codependency from the family member's perspective. Part II, The Family Recovery Program, describes this book's approach to family member recovery. Part III, Recovery Tools, describes the tools a recovery coach can use to aid a family member in their recovery process. The appendices have worksheets to help the family members understand the tools discussed in Part III. The appendices also have other valuable references for the recovery coach and family members.

PART I

SUD, Codependency and the Recovery Process

CHAPTER 2, Substance Use Disorder, Codependency, and Family Roles, discusses SUD, codependency, and family roles. The discussion in Chapter 2 gives the recovery coach the ability to discuss these topics with a family member so that the family member has both an intellectual and an emotional understanding of SUD, codependency, and family roles.

CHAPTER 3, The Family Member Recovery Process, takes the Substance Abuse and Mental Health Services Administration's (SAMHSA) guiding principle of recovery and stages of change and applies them to the family member recovery process.

CHAPTER 2

Substance Use Disorder, Codependency, and Family Roles

Ten years ago, the title of this chapter would have been "*Addiction, Codependency, and Family Roles.*" The publication of the fifth edition of the Diagnostic and Statistical Manual of Mental Disorders (DSM-5˚) changed the framework, the vocabulary, and the diagnostic criteria for problematic substance use. DSM-5˚ uses the term SUD and defines SUD in terms that are like those used for addiction. SUD is "...a cluster of cognitive, behavioral, and psychological symptoms indicating that the individual continues using the substance despite significant substance-related problems." (American Psychiatric Association 2013) SUD and addiction are not the same, however. SUD has three levels—mild, moderate, and severe. Severe SUD is comparable to the classic term addiction (McNeely and Adam 2020).

This book is going to refer to the DSM-5˚ approach to substance use. However, it will rely on the more traditional breakdown of substance use (e.g., experimentation, seeking, abuse/risky use, and addiction) and an adaptation of a relationship model developed by Nowinski (Nowinski 2011). This model describes the stages of SUD in terms of relationships (e.g., acquaintance, friend, committed relationship, enslavement). The traditional breakdown and the relationship models are used because these facilitate family members gaining a "head-understanding" and a "heart understanding" of SUD. Keep in mind that the DSM-5˙ breakdown of SUD was designed for clinicians to use when diagnosing a patient. It was not designed for recovery coaches, nor to give a family member an understanding of what their loved one is going through.

The terms codependent and codependency generate a good deal of controversy. Unlike SUD, the DSM-5˙ does not include codependency. This chapter discusses this controversy and provides a working definition of codependency that this book will use. The specific objectives of this chapter are to:

- Provide the information needed to discuss SUD with family members compassionately.

- Describe the progression of codependency in a manner that guides the help needed by the client.

- Understand the family roles often adopted by family members to respond to the SUD in the family.

The SUD section will discuss SUD's key concepts, methods to help family members understand these concepts, typical blocks to family member acceptance, and suggestions for moving past these blocks. The SUD section uses a relationship model of SUD that, in our experience, family members can more easily understand.

The codependency discussion uses a four-stage model developed by the authors to discuss the progression of codependency. When family members, especially parents/guardians, first seek help, they are usually coping through a combination of self-will and using the relationship tools they currently have. As the diseases of SUD and codependency progress, the family's everyday coping tools begin to fail. The stages of the codependency model provide a framework for where to focus your efforts.

The family roles section describes the typical behavior patterns the members of the SUD-burdened family adopt to cope with the turmoil caused by SUD. The purpose of discussing family roles is to allow the recovery coach to identify the coping mechanism the family member is using and provide appropriate assistance to transition the family member into recovery.

Substance Use Disorder

The SAMHSA definition of addiction makes it clear that SUD is a disease: "Addiction [severe SUD] is defined as a chronic, relapsing disorder characterized by compulsive drug seeking and use despite adverse consequences. It is considered a brain disorder because it involves functional changes to brain circuits involved in reward, stress, and self-control. Those changes may last a long time after a person has stopped taking drugs."[5] (National Institute on Drug Abuse 2020)

While family members are more familiar with the term "addiction," we recommend using SUD when talking to family members because it has several benefits. The first is that it emphasizes that SUD is a disease like many other diseases. Second, it avoids the many negative connotations society associates with the word addiction. Third, using SUD versus addiction makes it easier for the family member to gain a "heart" understanding that their loved one has a disease.

Assisting family members in gaining a "heart" understanding is essential because, in the beginning, family members either do not know or do not believe that SUD is a disease. This is usually not denial but a belief based on their own experience with substance use and the experience of friends and family. Many family members used substances and were able to control their substance use or stop when their substance use became problematic. In some cases, family members are currently responsibly using substances and cannot

---

5   This SAMHSA definition was taken from a website aimed at the general population. Addiction is in the definition because, unlike the four stages of cancer, the stages of SUD are not well known to the public.

understand why their loved one will not follow their example. Surprisingly, this is sometimes true for some family members recovering from SUD, especially if they were able to quit using substances on their own. Changing a family member's opinion on SUD is a slow process that requires constant education and patience. Attending support group meetings and hearing other family members' stories is the most effective method for gaining family member acceptance that SUD is, in fact, a potentially fatal disease.

STAGES OF SUD

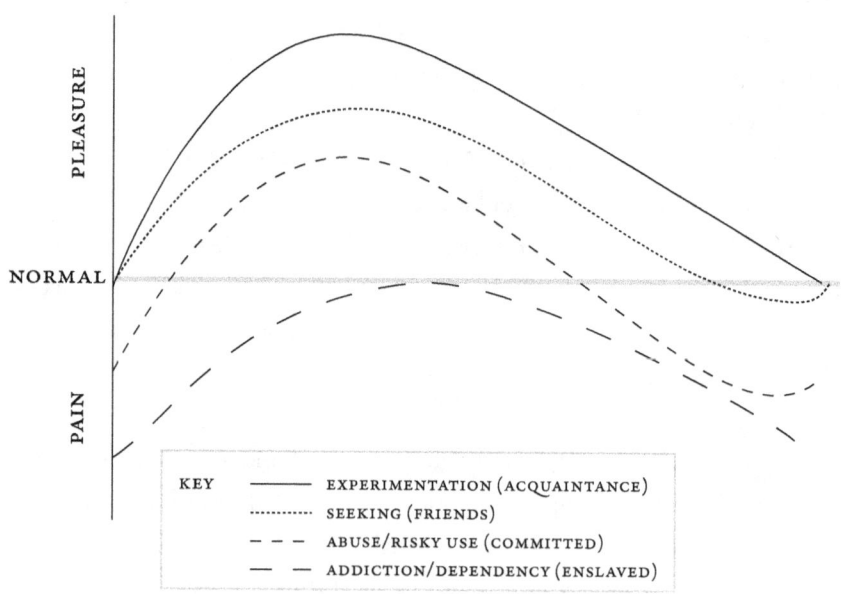

FIGURE 1. PLEASURE AND PAIN IN THE FOUR STAGES OF SUBSTANCE USE DISORDER

Figure 1 shows the four stages commonly used to describe the transition from just using a mind-altering substance to developing SUD as they relate to feeling normal, feeling pleasure, and feeling pain. It also shows the "relationship" counterpart to each stage of SUD.

Experimentation (Acquaintance)

The first is experimentation or first-use. Experimentation usually starts with a friend offering. The loved one accepts the offer sometimes as a way of relieving negative feelings (depression, anxiety, loneliness), a desire to feel good, a desire to fit in with the group, or out of an impulsive urge to try something regardless of the consequences (U.S. Department of Health and Human Services (HHS) 2016). As shown in the figure, during the experimentation phase, the person feels pleasure and returns to normal. Use continues because of the pleasurable feelings, and usually, there are no consequences. It is just fun.

The relationship in the experimentation phase is like an acquaintanceship. You do not see an acquaintance often and do not go out of your way to see them. If you see an acquaintance at a party, you might or might not say, "Hi." You will not go to a party just because the acquaintance is there, and you will not necessarily invite an acquaintance to your party. In the experimentation phase, use may or may not continue or become more frequent. At this point, the user can stop, and many do stop simply because it is illegal or because they do not like how it makes them feel.

Seeking (Friendship)

The next phase is the seeking phase. The loved one is making plans around drug use. The loved one will attend parties just because drugs will be there, and the loved one will avoid some parties because there will be no mind-altering substances. Use does not have to be every day, but it becomes regular (on weekends) or follows a set pattern—when depressed or anxious. As shown in *Figure 1*, substance use still results in pleasure but has negative consequences. The primary one is the unfulfilled desire to use substances again, but this desire is not overwhelming and does abate. Sometimes, the loved one overdoes it, and a hangover can result. In this phase, the loved one can control their substance use, and the loved one can stop if the consequences of drug use are severe enough.

In the seeking phase, the relationship is like a friendship. You will go to a party just because your friend is there. You will invite them to your parties, and you will spend time together with them. A friend can make you feel better when you are down, or you can have fun with them. You start wanting to be around them more. As with all friendships, you see your friend often but not every day. You miss them when you have not seen them for a while.

If your friend wants to do something illegal or dangerous, you might or might not go along. A friendship can end if something serious happens. Sometimes, a driving under the influence (DUI) arrest or an accident due to impaired driving will be enough for someone to stop or seriously cut back on their substance use. There is a sense of loss when the friendship ends, but it is not traumatic. In general, the user can quit using and may quit using, but it is more difficult to stop because the bond is more robust. A friendship can remain a friendship for an extended period or even a lifetime. People who can use substances normally ("normies") either stay in the "acquaintance" or "friendship" relationship. Approximately 8 percent of users progress to the last two types of relationships (U.S. Department of Health and Human Services (HHS) 2016).

Abuse/Risky Use (Committed Relationship)

An increased urge to use drives both substance abuse and risky substance use. Substance abuse is using more than needed, using unsafe combinations. Getting drunk is an excellent example of abusive substance use. Using substances in combination is another example of abuse. Abuse significantly increases the risk of an overdose. Risky use is also using substances in dangerous or unhealthy situations. Substance use before or while driving, substance use at school/work, and substance use before or during risky activities (skydiving, swimming, rock climbing, etc.) are good examples. Abuse/risky use is also characterized by continued use despite sometimes severe negative consequences—losing a job, divorce, impaired driving arrests, suspension from school, and failing grades.

Figure 1 shows the reason for abusive and risky use. When not using, there is pain and a strong urge to use. The person starts in pain and needs to use substances to first feel normal and then feel pleasure. Loved ones often describe this pain as deep depression or severe anxiety. Loved ones commonly say, "Using is the only thing that makes me feel normal." Unfortunately, depression and anxiety can be the result of their substance use. Substance use changed the biochemistry of the brain to the point that not having the substance generates feelings of unwellness that many call cravings.

The negative consequences are also more severe and more prolonged, but use continues because the craving is so intense. In this stage, emotional and mental changes become apparent; grades begin to drop, and behavioral problems start. Being late for work/school and aggressive behavior can start in this stage. Friends change, and legal issues begin (DUI, caught in possession). This is the stage of SUD where parents/guardians will start to seek help. In this stage, the user has almost lost the power of choice. A significant emotional event—DUI, loss of a spouse, overdose—can lead to a user stopping use.

Looking at abuse/risky use as a committed relationship—think unhealthy marriage—helps in understanding the continued use despite the consequences. Here, there is a genuine desire to keep the relationship. You want to be around the person daily. Prolonged periods of absence are difficult to bear. You can end the relationship, but the process and consequences are significant. Like a committed relationship, a person usually needs help to end the relationship. In marriage, it is legal help or therapy. For SUD, it is entering a recovery program that could include inpatient treatment.

Addiction/Dependency (Enslaved)

At this point, the user has lost the ability to stop and will continue to use substances despite severe consequences. The day begins with using and thoughts of use and ends with thoughts of using and using. Substance use has changed the brain to the point where the loved one believes that substance use is as essential for survival as breathing or eating. Tolerance and withdrawal are significant, and depending on the drug, withdrawal can be life-threatening. Recovery is possible and often requires inpatient treatment coupled with a long-term recovery program.

The drug has enslaved the loved one. Using and getting what is needed for the subsequent use are now the focus of the loved one's life. They have lost the ability to choose and have lost the ability to quit without significant assistance. Fortunately, the loved one always retains the ability to choose to enter recovery.

PARTING THOUGHTS ON SUD

Discussing SUD in terms of SUD's clinical and relationship models can help the family members identify where their loved one is in their drug use. Most of the families we worked with initially believed that their loved one was using substances occasionally. They thought this even though they were seeking help with what was happening in their family. Going through the stages and discussing them in terms of behaviors and relationships helps them to see what is going on with their loved ones. After discussing the progression of the disease, most family members were able to identify where their loved one was on the SUD spectrum.

The standard terms experimentation, seeking, abuse/risky use, and addiction/dependence illustrate both the progress of the disease and the seriousness of each of the stages. The relationship model helps the family member understand the feelings associated with drug use. Looking at the commitment change from an acquaintance to a friendship to an unhealthy marriage to enslavement is an understandable metaphor.

Both the clinical and relationship models help in understanding why it is so hard to quit in the later stages of SUD. A typical parent comment is, "I used drugs when I was in college, but when I graduated, I quit. Why can't he just quit?" The clinical model—changes in the brain—supplies the head-understanding. The relationship model provides the heart-understanding. Friendship is an almost universal experience, and parents have experienced committed relationships and either know how hard it is to leave these relationships or can imagine the difficulty. Family members and loved ones need both types of understanding.

The second benefit of this approach is that it humanizes the disease and the progression of the disease. This shift from clinical terms to humanistic ones helps family members remember that it is their loved one who has this disease. This relationship model illustrates how insidious the progression of the disease is by breaking it down into steps that readily relate to experiences family members have had. Few can pinpoint the moment or the event that transitioned an acquaintance into a friend or transitioned a friend into someone they loved and wanted to marry. Just like the person with SUD did not notice when their transitions occurred. This model humanizes the growing tenacity of the disease and relates to the increasing difficulty and the increasing pain associated with stopping substance use.

It is important not to shy away from or sugarcoat that addiction starts with the loved one choosing to use substances. For those under 21 years of age, this was an illegal and, in many traditions, immoral choice. In the first two stages of SUD, the loved one retains the ability to stop using. It is just as important to emphasize that using substances is *a necessary prerequisite for SUD*. Still, it is not the only factor that determines whether the loved one moves from normal use to contracting SUD. As already discussed, only a small percentage (8 percent) of users progress to contracting SUD (U.S. Department of Health and Human Services (HHS) 2016).

Codependency

The codependent or codependents are the family members that have taken on the role of trying to save the loved one. Codependency is a word that is difficult to define. Codependents Anonymous does not define the word but prefers to list the characteristics of codependency (Codependents Anonymous n.d.). Melody Beattie's definition is the closest one to what we see in family members, "A codependent person has let another person's behavior affect him or her, and who is obsessed with controlling that person's behavior" (Beattie 1992). Another standard description is someone who is addicted to the happiness of another person to the point that their own needs and wants, and other family members' needs and desires, do not matter. The American Psychological Association's *Dictionary of Psychological Terms* defines codependency as "a dysfunctional relationship pattern in which an individual is psychologically dependent on (or controlled by) a person who has a pathological addiction" (American Psychological Association 2023). This is the definition used in this book.

Many shy away from characterizing codependency as a disease and recommend not using the term because it is so ill-defined (Substance Abuse and Mental Health Services Administration 2020). However, treating codependency as a progressive disease is useful when working with family members because it relieves much of the stigma associated with codependency, and it aids in treating family members with the compassion needed for recovery (Lancer 2017). Codependency is often described as the disease of loving too much or helping too much.

SUD disrupts normal family processes because of the seriousness of the disease and how it adversely impacts each member of the family because of the steadily worsening behavior of the person with SUD. The loved one's behavior puts the loved one and the family at increasing emotional, relational, mental, physical, financial, and legal risk. This increased risk increases the ambient pain (e.g., anger, stress, anxiety, depression, mental illness) in the family. Without recovery, each family member develops their own coping mechanism, which is usually harmful or self-defeating. This section deals with one of the family member responses to SUD—codependency.

CODEPENDENCY

"During the most serious phase of my loved one's addiction, I was in the contradictory state of both being in denial and wanting to be the one who saved my loved one from addiction. I pictured my loved one coming to me later in life and saying, 'Dad, remember when you talked to me about getting sober, that was when my sobriety started.'

"I cannot believe I actually thought that, but I did. I was so guilty believing that I caused it that I wanted to be, needed to be the one that fixed it. Imagining that good feeling drove a lot of my enabling and false hope."

ANONYMOUS
FAMILYGROUP MEMBER

Many addiction professionals discuss codependency in terms of the phases of SUD. This approach implies that the progression of codependency is linked to the progression of SUD in the loved one. We have found that this is not always the case. Families can be in a crisis when their loved one is in SUD's experimentation (acquaintance) phase. Similarly, families can function well when the loved one is in the addiction/dependence (enslaved) phase. We have developed a four-stage model of codependency where we determine severity based on how well the family's self-will and current coping tools are keeping a good balance between the family feeling pleasure and pain. The authors developed the four stages based on their experience working with family members.

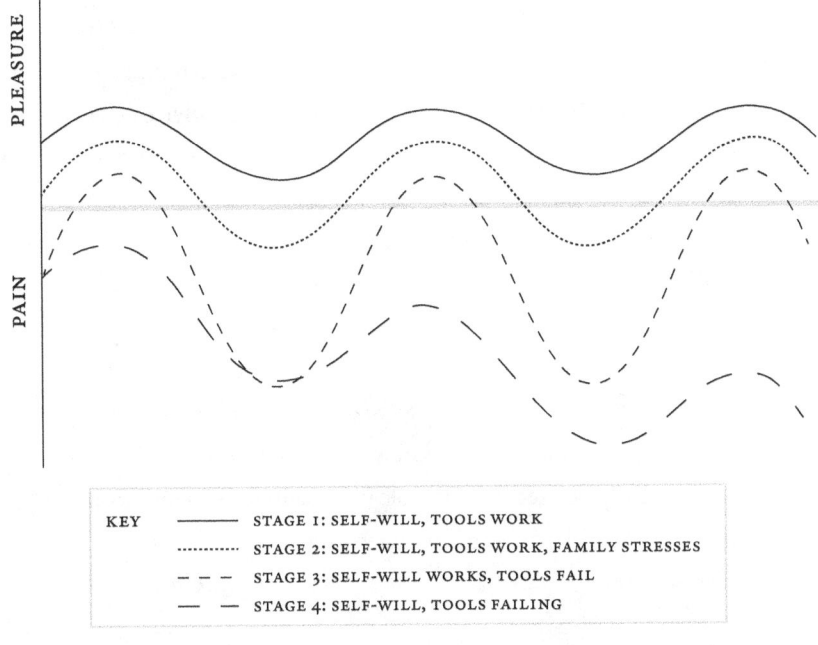

FIGURE 2. CODEPENDENCY'S PROGRESSION FROM NORMAL FAMILY FUNCTIONING TO CODEPENDENCY

Figure 2 is a graphic that illustrates the impact of codependency on family members in terms of feeling pleasure and feeling pain. The pain is a combination of fear, anger, anxiety, shame, guilt, and depression. The pleasure is a combination of satisfaction, enjoyment, accomplishment, and a general feeling of well-being. The progression depicted in *Figure 2* is without family members getting into recovery. Like SUD, recovery can change the course of codependency. We have divided the progression of codependency into four stages based on how the family's current relationship tools and self-will can maintain the balance between pleasure and pain.

WHAT IS SELF-WILL?

At this point, it is helpful to delve deeper into the concept of self-will. Merriam-Webster defines self-will as "The stubborn or willful adherence to one's desires and ideas. Obstinate" (Merriam-Webster 2023). A life based on self-will is destructive in recovery because it presupposes that we can manage our lives without needing a Higher Power or anyone's assistance or advice. Transitioning from a self-will-based life to a life willing to accept the wisdom of others and at least consider seeking God's will is a daunting task due primarily to a family member's life experiences. First, many family members successfully lived a life based on self-will. As Eric says,

> I knew I could solve the addiction in my family because I was known as the person to ask to solve complex problems. I could figure out almost anything. I knew I could find the solution on my own. I appreciated what people were saying in support group meetings, but I knew some of what they said was wrong, and the rest of what group members said did not apply to my family.

Second, learning to rely on a Higher Power's will requires having a trustworthy, benevolent Higher Power. Many family members do not have a Higher Power, do not trust their Higher Power, or their Higher Power was not really a Higher Power. Eric talks about his relationship with God (Eric's Higher Power) before recovery as more of a friendship. Sometimes, Eric needed God's help, and sometimes, God needed Eric's help. In the initial stages of his children's SUD, Eric did not want, nor did he think he needed God's help.

The problem with self-will is that it is a finite commodity, like the water in a water storage tank. A person's self-will tank can run dry, and unlike water storage tanks, you cannot replenish your self-will tank. Once it is gone, self-will is gone. Not surprisingly, failure is a significant drain on the self-will tank primarily because the self-will-driven person views the failure as their fault. Surprisingly, success also drains the self-will tank, but only a little. Even in success, some things could have gone better. The actual harm from self-will success is not the drain on the self-will tank but bolstering the belief that a person can live a self-will-directed life and be successful and happy. Multiple self-will successes will magnify the harm caused by a self-will failure. Eric is an excellent example of how success impacts self-will.

Eric's success before addiction in the family was the basis for his belief that he could solve the addiction problem. He studied hard in high school and was appointed to the United States Military Academy (West Point). He worked hard at West Point and earned a scholarship for a master's degree at a university of his choice. The Massachusetts Institute of Technology accepted Eric into its Nuclear Engineering master's program. The Army promoted Eric regularly. Eric earned a doctorate from the University of Pittsburgh. In Eric's mind, his actions and his choices were the reason for each of these successes. When his repeated attempts to cure his children's SUD or restore his marriage failed, Eric fell into what he describes as a bottomless dark pit and just wanted to give up. Giving up the arrogant reliance on self-will started Eric's real recovery.

In the detailed discussion of the stages of codependency below, self-will sustains a family member's codependency. When the self-will tank runs dry, the family member may start on a downward trajectory toward mental illness or substance use. Sometimes, this tank empties quickly and sometimes very slowly. Quickly or slowly, the sooner a family member enters recovery, the better.

STAGE 1: SELF-WILL AND FAMILY COPING TOOLS WORK

Every family has its homeostatic rhythm of life, of feeling well and not feeling well. As shown in *Figure 2*, this involves good times and tough times when the peaks are usually not too high, and the valleys are not too low. This is the normal state of affairs in a family where self-will and everyday relationship tools work. Each family member has their rhythm in this homeostatic environment. The family works to keep this rhythm constant, and the family usually can maintain a homeostatic rhythm during the experimentation/acquaintance phase of the loved one's SUD.

The family maintains its normal homeostasis during this stage primarily because the family does not know about the substance use or the substance use is within the bounds of the family norms. Some families accept underage alcohol use and underage marijuana use– not abuse. If family members do find out about uncondoned substance use or use that is outside the accepted norms, they will often ignore the reports, view it as a one-off, or not believe the reports. One client said his friends were telling him about his sister's drug use. His response was, "No way." He maintained his denial because his sister's behavior had not changed because she was only using substances occasionally. As her use continued and grew worse, her behavior changed and grew worse.

This is where substance use-related family conflicts can start primarily over how to respond to substance use that is outside family norms. However, it is unusual for a family to voluntarily seek help at this stage because their tools are generally working. The family is in its normal homeostatic cycle. Most families do not need help because substance use does not escalate to abuse/risky use, or addiction. For families, where the loved one's use, does escalate, not noticing use during this stage or noticing but not acting is a source of guilt, shame, and further arguments among family members.

STAGE 2: SELF-WILL AND FAMILY COPING TOOLS WORK, FAMILY IS UNDER STRESS

The loved one's substance use is now regular. Friends are changing, and the loved one's behavior is beginning to change. The family is noticing the changes. This is when the family's concern begins to elevate. The impact on the family depends on whether the substance use is legal or illegal, whether the substance user is an adult, an underaged (<21 years old) adult, or a minor. If the loved one is an adult, families often consider the use of legal substances in the seeking phase as normal. The family, especially a spouse, may start to feel slighted by the loved one because of the time the loved one is spending using substances, and they may not like the personality when the loved one is under the influence. The impact on the family of an adult using legal substances is usually minimal, and the family experiences tolerable shifts in its homeostasis. Self-will and the family's relationship tools are working, but there is increased tension in the family.

This changes if the loved one is a minor, an underaged adult, or an adult using illegal substances and the substance use is outside of the family norm.[6] Concern for the loved one increases in the family because of the legal liability of unlawful substance use, the potential impact on the loved one's future, and the physical danger associated with underage/illegal substance use. The most common family response is fear and shame, which the family usually expresses as anger or passive depression. The anger leads to shouting, shaming, and punishment. Passive depression leads to pleading, shaming, and desperate attempts to persuade the loved one to stop. Family members' resentment toward the loved one and the other family members increases. The codependent family members (usually the parents or guardians) begin to focus solely on the loved one.

---

6   Note that illegal substance use—usually underaged alcohol and marijuana use—is sometimes the norm in a family system.

Family members resent the loved one because of the disruption of the family caused by his/her substance use. Siblings begin to resent parents/guardians because the parents/guardians seem to be interested only in the loved one and ignore them. One family told the story of their son returning from college for summer break to find the house packed and ready for a move. The parents forgot about their son in college and neglected to tell him they were moving. The parents were moving in the hopes that their daughter would stop using substances once she was away from the "bad influences" in her life. It did not work.

Marriage issues and other relationship issues are beginning to surface with underage use or adult illegal drug use. Parents start to look for what caused the substance use and invariably blame themselves. At this point, the whole family begins to change to restore a new homeostasis to the family. Codependents move more into their codependency, and other family members move more into the roles they have adopted to cope. This new homeostasis has less pleasure and more anger, anxiety, and depression. This new homeostasis is manageable through self-will and the family's coping tools. Family members may or may not seek help in this phase. When the family seeks assistance, it is often court-ordered or a school requirement.

If the stress on the family from the loved one's drug use is decreased, the progression of codependency can stop or even be reversed. Family stress can be reduced under scenarios such as:

- An adult loved one does not progress past the seeking/friendship phase of substance use, and the substance use is acceptable to the family. In general, families may accept responsible alcohol use or responsible marijuana use where marijuana use is legal. It is much less likely that a family will accept illegal drug use.

- An underaged (<21 years old) minor or adult stops their illegal substance use.

- An adult loved one moves out.

STAGE 3: SELF-WILL IS WORKING; NORMAL RELATIONSHIP TOOLS ARE FAILING

Family members often describe this stage as a rollercoaster of highs and real lows. The loved one's drug use has progressed to the point where using substances is constant, and using is an essential part of their lives, just like a wife is an integral part of her husband's life. The family members are stressed and are beginning to focus more on their loved one. The family is starting to realize that their attempts to stop the loved one's substance use are not working. This is also where the family roles discussed in the next section become apparent. One parent said, "I just did what I always did when the tools did not work. I tried harder. I lectured longer. I yelled louder. I punished more. I just knew that it would work if I just found the right words, the right volume, the right punishment."

Enabling can temporarily relieve the codependent's misery in all stages, especially in this stage. Easing the loved one's pain by bailing them out of jail, replacing the totaled car, and not enforcing a boundary can bring the family pleasure and relief. Sometimes, family members view this kind of help as giving the loved one a fresh start and raising hopes. One dad relayed that he would give his loved one what they wanted because he wanted to feel the loved one's gratitude and see the smile on the loved one's face. This feeling of pleasure can lead to the family using enabling as a coping mechanism, and they can become reliant on enabling to relieve the pain. The joy of enabling makes the subsequent relapse or the following incident all the more painful.

The pain is so great because the tools are failing. In this stage, it is common for one or more family members to say, "I am the one keeping this family together. I need to keep it together." It gets harder and harder to "keep it together" as the loved one's behavior worsens. The loved one's violent outbursts in the home, stealing, dealing, constantly being under the influence, failing school, truancy, severe financial trouble, and extreme disruption of the family all serve to erode self-will. The energy needed to keep going when nothing is improving eventually overwhelms self-will, and they enter Stage 4.

STAGE 4: SELF-WILL FAILING AND NORMAL RELATIONSHIP TOOLS ARE FAILING

This is a debilitating stage for codependents and often occurs when the loved one is in the addiction/dependence/enslaved stage of SUD. At this point, the loved one's sole focus is using despite often catastrophic consequences. In this stage of SUD, the loved one's behavior often puts the family at risk. Family violence, keeping drugs in the home, dealing drugs, theft, being in risky situations, car accidents, and other criminal behavior generate both anger and concern born of fear in the family. The family member still gets relief from enabling—bailing out of jail, providing funds, providing transportation. The relief is short-lived because the help does not result in a change in drug use. At this stage, enabling can become almost addictive for the family member.

The codependent's sole focus at this point is fixing the loved one, and their efforts are not working. In this stage, tools have failed, the codependents' self-will has run out, and they have lost hope that their lives or their loved one's life will ever get better. This is where family members may check out and leave the family mentally or physically. This is also where marriages and other significant relationships are in serious jeopardy. In some cases, family members start having suicidal ideation because the pain is so unbearable. Despite all these adverse consequences, the family member's behavior will continue to deteriorate if the family member does not seek help.

PARTING THOUGHTS ON CODEPENDENCY.

It is important to remember that, like substance use, codependency is persistent because of the rewards felt by the codependent. Examples of these rewards include:

- **A FAMILIAR, COMFORTABLE WAY OF LIFE.** After a while, anxiety, self-pity, and anger become the usual way of life that the codependent is comfortable with. Recovery is a better way to live, but there is comfort in continuing to do what they have always done.

- **FOCUSING ON SOMEONE ELSE.** An ever-increasing focus on the loved one means the codependent does not need to focus on themselves and their issues. Similarly, this focus provides an excuse to avoid other problems with the rest of the family or in the codependent's significant relationships. There is great relief in having a good reason to avoid dealing with other thorny issues.

- **PROVIDING A COPING MECHANISM.** This is an important benefit for a codependent, and in many ways, the codependent needs this for recovery. The impact of a loved one with SUD on a family member can be emotionally catastrophic because of the family member's guilt. Guilt is generated by believing the family member caused SUD and is failing to control it. Entirely focusing on curing their loved one provides relief from guilt and shame.

- **MISERY PROVES HOW MUCH THE FAMILY MEMBER CARES ABOUT THE LOVED ONE.** Many family members come into recovery believing that loving the person with SUD meant the family member had to be anxious, had to sacrifice themselves for their loved one, and had to protect their loved one. Family members often express guilt over those times when the family member felt relief because their loved one was in treatment, in jail, or out of the house.

- **FEEL LIKE THE HERO.** The feelings of purpose, pride, courageousness, and satisfaction stemming from the belief that a family member is saving their loved one are powerful and difficult to combat. As one family member said, "For me, I also think I had a Superman complex about rescuing my daughter and got an endorphin rush from rescuing."

Each reward discussed above reinforces family members' belief that they are loving and caring. It should come as no surprise that early in recovery, a family member's first response to being told they are prideful, self-centered, and selfish is denial because what they are doing seems to be the opposite of these traits. Early in recovery, the second, more damaging response is to agree that they need to do better and then become more focused on their loved one, give more to the loved one, and try to become more of a martyr. Eric recalls the first time his sponsor told him he was prideful. Eric's response was, "No, I am not. I am the humblest person I know!" Think about that for a minute.

Whether you believe codependency is a progressive, relapsing mental disease or not, treating it as such will help both you and the family members you are working with. Treating it as a disease over which the client has no control can provide the separation needed to facilitate treating the codependent with the necessary compassion. Like the substance user, the codependent always has the choice to enter recovery. Still, they may not, and this is important, have the *ability* to stop enabling their loved ones until the recovery process provides them with the needed tools and support. The recovery coach's first job is to teach the recovery tools to the family member. The second job is to nurture the family member so they can realize they no longer need their harmful coping mechanism. Third, the recovery coach should encourage them to give up their non-recovery coping mechanism and use the recovery tools instead.

Needing something harmful seems counterintuitive, but it is not. A family member told a story of arguing with his wife for over a year and a half. Six months into the argument, he realized he knew exactly what to say to end it. He said, "I knew exactly what I needed to say to end the argument. I could not say it because I could not bear the thought of not having the anger. I still needed the anger to make it through the day. I continued working on my recovery, and the day finally came when the anger just left."

It is important to remember to be kind to the codependent and provide them with what they need at the moment. The urge to save loved ones and the urge not to feel the pain of losing a loved one are powerful motivators to continue trying desperately to rescue their loved one. Like the loved one, it sometimes takes feeling the consequences of codependency to prod a family member into recovery. Like the loved one, a codependent often must hit a personal bottom to move into recovery. It is often difficult for a coach to watch a family member undergo this process. One father described his bottom: "All I ever wanted out of life was a happy marriage and a good family. I was in my backyard sitting on a tree swing when I realized that I was losing my marriage and my family, and everything I tried was not working. I was desperately despondent and depressed. My real recovery started when I truly recognized my powerlessness."

Family Roles

Families are a system. The family needs security, acceptance, warmth, humor, a sense of belonging, and pride. Each member of the family has a role in providing these. Like any other system, families want to reach a state of homeostasis that works for the family as a whole. When one member of the family changes, the rest of the family adapts to that change to try to meet the basic family needs, if it is a minor, standard change—such as joining the military, leaving for college, starting a new job, etc.—the family can adjust and continue. A significant change - such as a death, someone contracting a major illness, divorce, etc.—can lead to drastic unhealthy changes in the family. Families with SUD change, and family members adopt distinct roles to cope with the potentially lethal change in the family. SAMHSA's Treatment Improvement Protocol (TIP) 39, *Substance Use Disorder and Family Therapy* breakdown of family roles, is the basis for this family roles discussion (Substance Abuse and Mental Health Services Administration 2020).

The purpose of the Family Roles section is to provide an understanding of how different family members cope with the SUD in the family. It is important to understand that the loved one's SUD has deeply affected the family, which led to the family members adopting coping mechanisms that help them and the rest of the family. The coping mechanism often involves adopting one or a couple of the below-mentioned roles. The first key point is that the family member does not need to stay in these roles but can recover to become an integrated whole person. The second is that, without help, each family member can have serious mental health issues.

The roles outlined are generalizations of family members' responses to SUD in the family. The family roles explain, in part, why the codependents, usually guardians/parents, begin to focus all their attention on the loved one. The hero seems to have it all together, doing well in everything. The mascot is funny and joking around. The lost child is never an issue because they keep to themselves. The scapegoat acts out to get attention, however undesirable the attention is. However, these family members also need help to recover. They can also get to the point where mental illnesses and suicide may occur. Recovery coaches usually work with parents/guardians, but the other family members also need the recovery support a recovery coach provides. The 12-Step process supported by recovery coaches and family group meetings is effective in helping every member of the family.

LOVED ONE (SUBSTANCE USER)

As already said, we refer to the person with SUD as the loved one. The loved one is also called the addict, the victim, or the dependent. The characteristics of the loved one depend on where they are on the SUD scale. As substance use increases, the loved one becomes more self-centered, and the rest of the family becomes more centered on the loved one. The loved one becomes the focus of the family. Unsurprisingly, the one statement heard often from the loved one is, "If you all would just leave me alone, I would be fine."

Two dynamics are in play with the loved one. First, as the disease progresses, the loved one's dependence on the drug increases to the where the loved one needs to use substances just to be able to live in their skin. At this point, substance use has rewired the brain to believe that survival requires using substances. Anything that blocks this substance use is a threat to the loved one's survival. Second, the loved one has a powerful sense of denial that stops them from admitting that they have become dependent on the substance. Both dynamics lead to the loved one:

- **DENYING THEY HAVE A PROBLEM AND BLAMING EVERYONE ELSE FOR THEIR DRUG USE.** "I am using because my parents are so controlling." "I need to use it because my life is so bad." "They do not understand the drug is the only thing that makes me feel good." Finally, "I need to use, or I will die. They do not understand."

- **LASHING OUT IN ANGER AND FRUSTRATION.** This occurs especially if the family tries to curtail substance use or refuse to enable substance use or refuse to shield them from the consequences of their substance use. The family setting and enforcing boundaries also triggers anger and frustration.

- **BECOMING VERY MANIPULATIVE AND CAN BECOME VERY CHARMING.** This, especially for teenagers, is normal. SUD amplifies this because of the increasing strength of the urge to use. After getting sober, a loved one said, "When I wanted something from my parents, I would first ask nicely. If they refused, I would get angry. If they still refused, I would start crying. The crying usually worked."

- **FILLED WITH SELF-PITY AND EVENTUALLY SELF-LOATHING.** Denial that their substance use is an issue coupled with denial that they are responsible for the consequences leads to a good deal of self-pity. These things are happening to them versus they are happening because of their choices and actions.

On the inside, our loved ones are filled with shame, guilt, fear, pain, and hurt. The loved one can return to an everyday, productive life with recovery. Without recovery, the outcomes are usually either prison or premature death.

THE CODEPENDENT (CARETAKER, ENABLER)

The codependent is often called the primary caretaker, martyr, or chief enabler. This is the person who is trying to hold the family together by attempting to make the loved one stop using, protecting the loved one from the consequences of their drug use, and protecting the family from the loved one. The statement heard most often from the codependent is, "If you would just stop using, the family would be fine."

The codependent becomes focused on the loved one as the loved one becomes focused on substances. The codependent cares. They care about their loved one, and they care about their family. As the family disease progresses, the codependent begins to feel helpless, unable to make decisions, and may develop substance use issues or mental health issues. Sometimes, the codependent becomes addicted to caretaking, and they feel an overwhelming impulse to control and to try to fix things. Eventually, the codependent can lose all sense of self, self-worth, and self-care as they continue to focus on the loved one.

Like the loved one, the codependent needs a recovery plan to pull them out of their "addiction" and allow them to lead a valuable, productive life. Without recovery, the codependent can become a substance abuser, suffer from mental illness, lose a sense of self, withdraw from society, and become truly angry and bitter. (It is important to remember the substance user needs at least one enabler to keep using.)

THE HERO

The hero brings pride and a sense of worth to the family. The hero copes with the family dysfunction and the shame of being "that family"[7] by doing everything possible to succeed at whatever they do. Typically, the hero is the one who works hard at school and participates in multiple activities. Other characteristics of the hero may include the following:

- **THE HERO CAN BECOME OBSESSED WITH SUCCESS.** This obsession can get to the point where they become workaholics who tie their self-worth to their success at work. Eventually, the hero views even minor setbacks as catastrophic failures that may lead to extreme anxiety, depression, and even suicide.

- **THE HERO'S SUCCESS CAN LEAD TO BELIEVING THEY CAN AND SHOULD CONTROL OUTCOMES.** This belief leads them to try to control other people. The hero takes it especially hard when they fail, or other people do not do things the way they want them done.

- **THE HERO CAN BELIEVE THEY ARE DOING EVERYTHING FOR THE FAMILY AND NO ONE ELSE IS HELPING.** This can lead to a feeling of being used and eventually anger at the family. The hero is mad at the loved one for causing the family dysfunction. The hero is angry at the primary caretaker for not fixing the loved one and saddling the hero with so much responsibility.

---

7 '...that family." The family in the neighborhood that everyone talks about, usually in disparaging terms, because of the SUD in the family.

Like the loved one and the codependent, the hero needs a recovery plan to pull them out of their "addiction" and allow them to lead a valuable, productive life. Without recovery, the hero can become a workaholic or substance abuser, suffer from mental illness, lose a sense of self, withdraw from the family, and become incredibly angry and bitter.

THE SCAPEGOAT

"I hate this family! I am out of here!" The scapegoat is the member of the family who may see clearly what is going on in the family but becomes frustrated that no one is listening to them. No one is paying attention to them because the family is focused on the loved one. The only way the scapegoat can get attention is to act out. They may begin to act out either out of frustration ("Doesn't anyone see what is going on!") or out of neglect ("Doesn't anyone see me!"). In many respects, the scapegoat diverts attention from the loved one and the other members of the family by acting out. Sometimes, the family blames the scapegoat for the loved one's substance use. Other characteristics of the scapegoat may include the following:

- **THE SCAPEGOAT CAN BECOME ANGRY, BITTER, AND FRUSTRATED.** Angry, upset, and frustrated that no one else is willing to admit what is going on, and, in some instances, the family is falsely blaming them for the turmoil in the family.

- **THE SCAPEGOAT CAN FEEL OSTRACIZED.** Like the loved one, the family is excluding the scapegoat. Unlike the loved one, no one pays attention to the scapegoat.

Without recovery, the scapegoat can become a substance abuser, suffer from mental illness, lose a sense of self, withdraw from society, withdraw from the family, and become angry and bitter. With recovery, they can lead productive, fulfilling lives.

THE MASCOT

The mascot deals with the family's tension and dysfunction by adding comic relief. The mascot is the jokester and uses humor to diffuse arguments or awkward moments. Outwardly, the mascot is okay. They appear cute, immature, fun-loving, laughing, and telling jokes. Inside, the mascot is lonely, fragile, fearful, and insecure.

Without recovery, the mascot can become a substance abuser, suffer from mental illness, lose a sense of self, withdraw from society, withdraw from the family, and become truly angry and bitter. With recovery, they can lead productive, fulfilling lives.

THE LOST CHILD

The lost child relieves the family because they are withdrawn and do not cause trouble. The lost child is the forgotten child that is inwardly focused. They are shy and quiet and do not get into trouble. They attach to things or pets rather than people. They tend to avoid stress or conflict, and they have few friends. They are often the child that the family forgets to talk about or the child that the family forgets their birthday.

The lost child feels rejected, lonely, unimportant, and anxious. This can lead to depression, anxiety, obsessive-compulsive disorder, substance use, or, in the extreme, suicide. All of this can go unnoticed because they are not causing trouble. With recovery, they can lead productive, fulfilling lives.

PARTING THOUGHTS ON FAMILY ROLES

The main takeaway from the family roles is that each family member needs help. The person with SUD needs help to prevent potentially catastrophic outcomes. It is less obvious, but true, that every family member also needs help to avert less desirable, if not disastrous, consequences. When talking to a family member, it helps to ask about other family members. Often, the parent/guardian is so focused on the loved one that you will never hear about their other children in support group meetings or an appointment unless you ask them directly. You might hear about the scapegoat, the one that is acting out. It is unlikely that parents/guardians will discuss the hero, the mascot, or the lost child because they are not "causing trouble." They are not causing trouble, but, more than likely, they are in trouble.

These roles are presented to ensure recovery coaches can better see the hurt masked by the mascot's joking, the hero's "I have it together," and the lost child's compliant distance. It is important to remember that each family member feels isolation, shame, and guilt; unconditional acceptance and unconditional love can ameliorate these feelings. Like the codependent and the loved one, it is common for family members not to want nor to believe that they do need help.

One way to break through these defense mechanisms is an invitation to an activity. Our organizations routinely have a *Talent-No-Talent* show. We do this both for fun and healing. It is common for a recalcitrant family member to either come to or participate in the event and eventually become a part of the group. This is especially true for teen siblings and pre-teen siblings. Many a "star" was born at this event.

Be very alert for signs of mental illness in these family members, especially the hero and the lost child. These two can seem to have it together and may, but their need for help can be genuine.

CHAPTER 3

The Family Member Recovery Process

Chapter 2 discussed how the loved one, the codependent, and the rest of the family progress without a recovery program. This chapter examines the essential components or principles of the recovery process as defined by SAMHSA and the stages of change described by Prochaska (Substance Abuse and Mental Health Services Administration, 2013; Prochaska JO, 1992) from the perspective of a family member. Both the principles of recovery and the stages of change were developed for the loved one with SUD, but they also apply to a family member's codependency. The objectives of this chapter are to:

- Provide a practical understanding of the SAMHSA guiding principles of recovery as they apply to family members.

- Describe the stages of change.

- Demonstrate how a peer recovery coach can use the recovery principles and stages of change to work with family members more effectively.

SAMHSA's guiding principles, the stages of change, and how to apply them to a family member's recovery are all important. The recovery coach needs a good understanding of these concepts to shepherd a family member through their unique recovery process effectively.

Guiding Principles of Recovery

The principles of recovery used in this book are based on the SAMHSA pamphlet entitled *SAMHSA's Working Definition of Recovery: 10 Guiding Principles of Recovery* (Substance Abuse and Mental Health Services Administration 2012). The SAMHSA pamphlet sets three objectives for recovery from SUD—attain health and wellness, live a self-directed life, and attain a life that maximizes their potential. SAMHSA categorized the resources needed to support recovery into four recovery supports—health, home, purpose, and community. Health includes the resources necessary to address all aspects of physical health, mental health, and well-being. "Home" consists of a safe, stable home and resources needed to meet physical needs—food, clothing, and transportation. "Purpose" addresses what brings meaning to life—a job, education, meaningful activities, and the resources (income, transportation, independence) needed to live a consequential life. "Community" is the relationships and social networks that provide acceptance and nurturing.

Recovery capital is another framework for describing the resources needed for recovery. Recovery capital divides these resources into four distinct categories—social capital, physical capital, human capital, and cultural capital (Cloud and Granfield 2008). SAMHSA's resource categorization and recovery capital differ, but each has the same essential components. We are using SAMHSA's guiding principles for the basis of this book because they also include the elements of recovery capital. Please see Cloud and Granfield (Cloud and Granfield 2008) or White and Cloud (White and Cloud 2008) for a more detailed discussion of recovery capital.

SAMHSA's guiding principles and recovery capital briefly refer to spirituality but do not treat spirituality or a belief in a Higher Power as a necessary building block for recovery. In both the 12-Step approach and the approach used in this book, spirituality is the fundamental building block for recovery, *especially for family members*. For this reason, this section discusses the importance of spirituality as a guiding principle in recovery.

RECOVERY IS SUPPORTED BY SPIRITUALITY

Spirituality has different meanings for different people and in different cultures. Dr. Maya Spencer authored an article on spirituality for the Royal College of Psychiatrists website that captured the essence of spirituality in a 12-Step context. Dr. Spencer defined spirituality as "...the recognition of a feeling or sense that there is something greater than myself [sic], something more to being human than sensory experience, and that the greater whole of which we are a part is cosmic or divine in nature" (Spencer 2012). One of the goals of a 12-Step program is to strengthen a recovering person's spiritual connection with their Higher Power so they can hear and align themselves with God's will. The 12 Steps accomplish this realignment by guiding the recovering person to pursue each spiritual value that infuses the 12 Steps. *Table 1* below has the spiritual values the authors associated with each of the 12 Steps.

TABLE 1. SPIRITUAL VALUES FOR EACH OF THE 12 STEPS

Step	Spiritual Values	Step	Spiritual Values
Step 1	Acceptance, Humility	Step 7	Humility, Faith
Step 2	Hope	Step 8	Willingness, Honesty, Courage
Step 3	Faith	Step 9	Agape Love, Courage, Faith
Step 4	Courage, Forgiveness	Step 10	Integrity, Perseverance
Step 5	Honesty, Courage	Step 11	Self-discipline, Faith, Submission
Step 6	Patience, Humility	Step 12	Service

RECOVERY EMERGES FROM HOPE

Re-instilling hope is one of the first tasks for a coach because a family usually asks for help when they have lost hope for their loved one's recovery. Regaining hope for a family member is a two-stage process. First, the family member regains the hope that their loved one can recover. Second, the family member regains the hope that they can regain their lives whether or not their loved one recovers. Attending group meetings, attending individual appointments, participating in activities, and working the 12 Steps all foster hope and the mental and emotional resilience hope provides. The relief this program brings reinforces the family member's hope. The program brings relief through unconditional love, unconditional acceptance, a focus on spirituality, and an emphasis on having fun.

RECOVERY IS PERSON-DRIVEN

Like the loved one, the family member manages their recovery. They set their recovery process, set their own recovery goals, and develop their plan for achieving them. Solving their problems instills a sense of control over their lives, and fosters hope for the future. In many ways, this helps the 11th promise of Alcoholics Anonymous (AA) come true for family members: "We will intuitively know how to handle situations that used to baffle us." The coach's task is to provide the information, the encouragement, and the accountability needed for a family member to make informed recovery decisions. We are not about changing people's lives. We are about giving people the recovery tools to make the necessary changes in their lives.

Family members are often hesitant to start a recovery program. The most common statement is, "I do not have a problem. My loved one has a problem." Education can help overcome this, but more than anything, going to support group meetings and hearing stories is the catalyst that moves a family member into recovery. Family members are responsible for their recovery, but their recovery requires the help of the group and others in recovery. This is a "We" program.

RECOVERY OCCURS VIA MANY PATHWAYS

There are many effective pathways to recovery for family members. Our approach is the 12-Step approach augmented with individual recovery coaching. Within the 12-Step framework, there are multiple pathways to recovery because each person starts recovery with different pasts (including past trauma), talents, dislikes, cultures, beliefs, personalities, life goals, character defects, and character strengths. An individual family member's recovery path may include only attending support group meetings, or it may consist of recovery coaching, meetings, working with a sponsor, activities, and therapy. The uniqueness of every family member highlights the importance of meeting our clients where they are without preconceived notions of what their recovery path ought to be.

Not surprisingly, everyone's recovery path has both periods of growth and setbacks. A relapse for a family member is falling back into their codependent behaviors. This usually occurs when their loved one relapses or must face dire consequences. Like a SUD relapse, a family member's relapse can occur at any time during their recovery. Both substance use and non-substance use-related issues can trigger a family member's relapse.

RECOVERY IS HOLISTIC

Holistic recovery recognizes first that all aspects of a person's life can contribute to or hinder recovery. The 12-Step world categorizes holistic recovery in terms of mind, body, and spirit. The SAMHSA classifies holistic support in terms of its recovery supports—health, home, purpose, and community. The authors believe these are not conflicting approaches to holistic recovery but complementary. We recommend using all seven when working with family members.

RECOVERY IS SUPPORTED BY PEERS AND ALLIES

Peer support is fundamental for 12-Step recovery programs for loved ones and family members. For family members, peers provide understanding, acceptance, sympathy, and empathy. This peer environment offers a safe place for family members to share what is going on in their lives. In support group meetings or appointments with peer recovery coaches, you can see family members' relief when they realize that peer coaches and the people in our meetings understand what the family member is going through because they have been there.

Allies—therapists, psychologists, psychiatrists, child protective services, adult protective services, and the justice system—are just as important for family members as they are for the loved one with SUD. Family members also have any number of mental health issues that may require therapy and therapeutics. Often, family members have suffered severe trauma in their lives and will need the help of specialists. The stress added by the loved one can be so extreme that the family requires child protective services, adult protective services, or law enforcement services.

RECOVERY IS SUPPORTED THROUGH RELATIONSHIPS AND SOCIAL NETWORKS

Family members dealing with SUD often become isolated from friends, community organizations, social circles, and faith-based communities. Some of the isolation is self-imposed by the shame/guilt the family member feels. Family members may be afraid to venture out because they are too shame/guilt-ridden and afraid of others judging them. Some of the isolation is from external sources. Well-meaning community members offer conflicting advice based on a misunderstanding of SUD and its impact on the family. Often, the community will shun the family because of ignorance of the disease and the stigma of addiction. This isolation worsens the family member's anxiety, depression, fear, and codependency.

Pulling oneself out of isolation requires the support of peers and the development of a social network with people who will enable recovery. This is the "stick with winners" principle, where a "winner" is a person, social group, or organization that enables the family member's recovery. Peers in recovery enable recovery. Organizations like Al-Anon, Nar-Anon, Parents of Addicted Loved Ones, RecoveryWerks!, and PDAP enable family member recovery. Winners, peers, and recovery organizations give family members a sense of relief, belonging, sanity, safety, fellowship, and happiness that are vital for family member recovery.

RECOVERY IS CULTURALLY BASED AND INFLUENCED

Families can live in three, sometimes synchronous, sometimes asynchronous cultures. The first is the society they are living in. The United States has a distinct yet eclectic culture that is a composite of our founding culture and the cultures of those who immigrated to the U.S. The second is their heritage-based culture. Italian culture differs from Nigerian, Hispanic, African-American, and Chinese cultures. Then, the culture of the family itself. Each family has its unique micro-culture. Effective recovery coaching must align with the individual's culture in each context, especially the context of the family's micro-culture. We can study and learn about the societal culture and the heritage culture. However, we can only learn about the family's micro-culture and the individual's culture by building trusting relationships. Basing coaching only on the heritage culture runs the risk of being culturally insensitive to the individual's specific culture. Individual recovery needs to be based on the individual.

RECOVERY IS SUPPORTED BY ADDRESSING TRAUMA

Like people with SUD, family members may have past or current trauma. In general, a recovery coach is not trained to address trauma, but they are trained to provide trauma-informed care for family members. Trauma-informed care includes creating a safe environment, understanding the warning signs that the client may need a higher level of care, and supplying the resources the client requires (Substance Abuse and Mental Health Administration 2014). It is also helpful to know how to respond to a past trauma-induced crisis. It is common for repressed trauma to emerge when a family member is in recovery. Often, the coach or other family members will be aware of the trauma before the individual with the trauma is aware. Dealing with emerging repressed trauma requires the help of a trauma-trained professional. Once the recovery coach suspects suppressed trauma, it is essential to refer the family member to mental health professionals trained in trauma treatment.

RECOVERY INVOLVES INDIVIDUAL, FAMILY, AND COMMUNITY STRENGTHS AND RESPONSIBILITY

Family members often lose the ability to stop enabling, just like the loved one with SUD has lost the power of choice over their substance use. However, both the family member and the loved one retain the power to choose to enter recovery. The importance of family member recovery for both the family member and the individual with SUD is well documented. SAMHSA TIP 39, *Substance Use Disorder Treatment and Family Therapy,* has an excellent summary of the scientific literature on the connection between family recovery and the loved one's recovery[8] (Substance Abuse and Mental Health Services Administration 2020).

---

8   TIP 39 does not directly address the benefits of family member recovery to the family member. This is a shortcoming in the TIP as well as in the general literature on recovery.

The community is responsible for providing the environment in which recovery can flourish. This includes provision of recovery resources, provision of prevention resources, and community-wide education. The community also has the responsibility to create a social environment where two contradictory norms exist: the community views substance abuse[9] as socially unacceptable, and the community views a person with SUD as a person who needs compassion and treatment. This may seem like a daunting task, but it has already been done for tobacco-induced cancer and Type II diabetes. Tobacco use is discouraged. People living with tobacco-induced cancer receive treatment and are treated with compassion. The same is true for Type II diabetes patients who do not follow prescribed diets and exercise regimens. Yes, there are differences. SUD is associated with increased family distress, violence, and crime. These differences are not insurmountable, as shown by the general increase in accepting SUD as a disease.

RECOVERY IS BASED ON RESPECT

Coaches/counselors respect the family members as they respect themselves. Respecting a person does not mean agreement with their beliefs or actions. It does mean honoring the person's right to choose and follow their own path; respecting the person includes protecting their civil rights and their right to believe as they choose to believe. Respect also includes providing family members with the tools to learn how to respect themselves first and then to respect those around them.

PARTING THOUGHTS ON THE SAMHSA PRINCIPLES

Neither SAMHSA's four recovery supports nor their guiding principles specifically include spirituality. The authors added spirituality to SAMHSA's principles

---

9   Substance abuse includes the use of illegal substances, the abuse of legal substances and all underage substance use.

because of the importance of spirituality in most, if not all, recovery pathways. Please notice that the term is spirituality and not religion. The 12 Steps do not require a belief in God. The 12 Steps require a belief in a power greater than us. For some family members, it is the group. For some, their Higher Power is reason, logic, or science. It is important to remember that spirituality is as important for family members as it is for the person trying to stop using substances.

The second principle—recovery emerges from hope—is the most important for family members in early recovery. Most family members seek help when they have lost hope. They can express their hopelessness in anger, self-pity, depression, frustration, disinterest, and anxiety. The root of all of this is hopelessness. First-contact with a family member is about giving them hope. Yes, there is the hope that their loved one can recover, but also hope that they can get their lives back whether their loved one chooses recovery or not. This sounds like an impossible task, but it is not. Simple things like laughter in an appointment, complimenting them on something they did correctly, giving them simple boundaries, and relaying parts of your story can provide hope that hope can be restored.

Often, family members are on different, sometimes conflicting paths. Attempting to reconcile these differences is the first step; however, sometimes, the differences are irreconcilable. The following happened to two couples. In both cases, their adult son relapsed, and the boundary was that a relapse meant their sons could not remain in the home. For both couples, one parent wanted to enforce the boundary, and the other did not. Since both parents owned the house, the son could legally stay if one parent allowed him to stay. Each couple took different approaches to managing this conflict.

In the first couple, the wife did not want to enforce the boundary, but the husband did. The husband decided to accept something he could not control—his wife allowing the son to stay in the home. He also developed boundaries for both his wife and his son. The second couple was the reverse. The husband did not want to enforce the boundary, and the wife did. Living with her using-son was something the wife could not accept, so she moved out of the house until their son voluntarily left years later. Both couples, as of this writing, are still together. Both couples worked on their own recovery programs.

Family Member Stages of Change

The Prochaska stages of change (*Figure 3*) for recovering from SUD are also applicable to a family member's recovery from codependency (Prochaska JO 1992). In precontemplation, the family member does not believe they need help. Like the loved one, the family member can be in any one of the four stages of codependency and still not think they need help. In contemplation, the family member is open to getting into recovery. In the preparation stage, they have decided to enter recovery and are developing a recovery plan. The action step is the implementation of the plan. In the maintenance phase, family members continue to use their recovery tools. Like their loved ones, family members can relapse into codependent behaviors. What follows is a more detailed discussion of each stage of change.

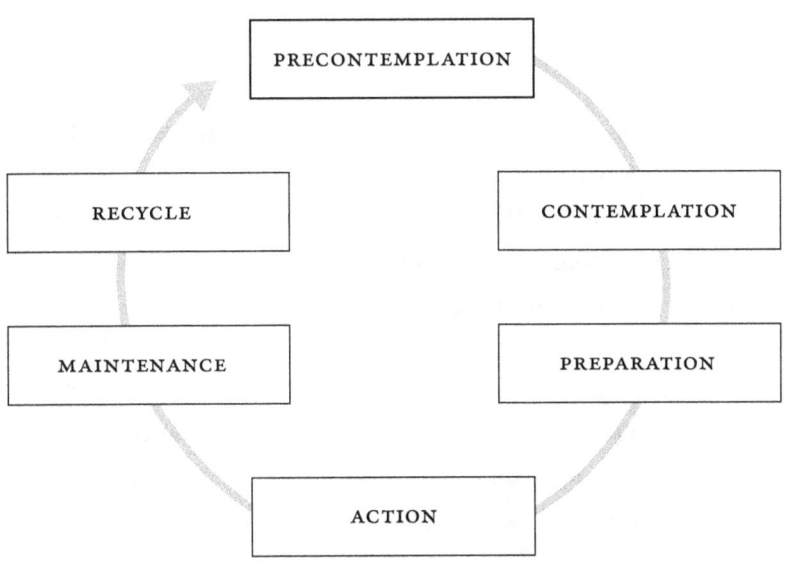

FIGURE 3. STAGES OF CHANGE FOR RECOVERING FROM SUD AND CODEPENDENCY

PRECONTEMPLATION

In the precontemplation stage of change, the family member does not believe they need help. In this phase, the family member may not participate in the program at all or take part only as a show of support for their loved one or another family member (e.g., a husband attending to support his wife). There are multiple reasons for this that range from not believing it is a disease to just not thinking they need help. Family members in this stage often say, "It is just a phase." "My loved one needs help. I do not need help." "Just fix them, and all will be well." "I am here just for support." "I am here just because the court/school is making me attend." Left on their own, family members in precontemplation will not seek help until the situation at home is unbearable (Stage 2, 3, or 4 codependence) or the legal/school system intervenes and mandates parent and loved one attendance at support group meetings.

CONTEMPLATION

The family member acknowledges this is a new problem and needs help. The family member may not be sure that a 12-Step recovery program will work for them, but they are usually open to hearing about 12-Step recovery. In this stage of change, it is common for family members to want to learn how to "fix" their loved one. Common characteristics include:

- **THEY HAVE A DESPERATE DESIRE TO FIX THEIR LOVED ONE AND DO NOT KNOW HOW TO PROCEED.** A desperate need to save a loved one usually drives the family member's willingness to begin a recovery program.

- **THEY ARE SKEPTICAL THAT THIS APPROACH WORKS.** This is especially true for people from family-centric cultures where family opinions and traditional child-rearing methods are highly valued.

- **THEY DO NOT RECOGNIZE THAT RECOVERY IS ABOUT THEM CHANGING.** It often takes a while for the family member to realize that they are working a program for themselves and not for their loved one. A statement often heard in meetings about this is, "I came here for my loved one. Now I know I am here for me."

In this stage, it is essential to give encouragement and meet the family member where they are. Other helpful actions include:

- **USE MOTIVATIONAL INTERVIEWING.** In general, motivational interviewing can move a client from ambivalence about the need for change to wanting to change to developing a plan to attain the desired change. Motivational interviewing is in line with our approach because it is client-based. The client names their motivation for change. The client develops their change plan. The coach's role is to help this process. Miller and Rollnick's book, *Motivational Interviewing: Helping People Change*, discusses the motivational interviewing process in detail (Miller and Stephen 2013).

- **DISCUSS CODEPENDENCE KINDLY.** Like a loved one, shaming or manipulating a family member to get help usually does not work. When it does work, the family member usually resists the more difficult actions—getting a sponsor or enforcing a boundary. A good approach is to discuss recovery as a process of getting a new set of relationship tools. A father in the program put it this way, "My wife and I had five children. Our parenting tools worked for the first three. Our tools also worked for our youngest two until they became addicted. We needed new parenting tools, and recovery gave us those tools."

- **STRESS HOPE AND COMMUNITY.** Hope and the understanding that they are not alone anymore are two of the most important gifts a coach can give a family member. Knowing there is a community of safe people who understand what they are going through can bring a family member "in from the cold." Hope comes from knowing there is a way out of the turmoil the family is experiencing.

PREPARATION

In the preparation stage, the client wants to change, and with the coach's aid, they develop a recovery plan. This can be a written plan or a discussion of the next steps. It is helpful to encourage a written plan. Chapter 8, Family Member Recovery Plan, has more information on developing a family member recovery plan.

ACTION

In the action step, the family member implements a formal or informal recovery plan. Boundaries are set and often enforced. This is also where the family member usually gets a sponsor, attends support group meetings regularly, and has regular appointments with their coach. This is a critical time for family members because they are changing themselves, which is hard, but they are also changing how they interact with their family and friends. Some, especially their loved ones, will not like the changes. Actions the recovery coach can take to support a family member in early recovery include:

- **CONTINUE RELATIONSHIP DEVELOPMENT.** Continue developing and nurturing the coaching relationship with the client. Provide hope by reminding the client of past victories, sharing personal stories, and relating the successes of other clients. Providing hope is especially important after a loved one's relapse or a codependent relapse.

- **PROVIDE EDUCATION ON RECOVERY TOOLS.** Teach the client the recovery tools to support their recovery. This is the time to teach the client about boundaries, living in the moment, and recovery beliefs. Part II of this book provides recovery tools for family members.

- **PROVIDE ASSISTANCE THAT IS CONSISTENT WITH THE SCOPE OF A RECOVERY COACH.** This includes assisting in getting the loved one advanced care when needed, helping with obtaining financial aid, recommending mental health specialists, and assisting in finding housing. The focus here is helping the family members find the resources they need.

- **PROVIDE ENCOURAGEMENT, PRAISE, AND CONFRONTATION.** Major changes occur in the action stage of recovery that can be daunting. Encouraging change and praising changes when they occur are important. Equally important is lovingly confronting a client when they are off course.

MAINTENANCE

This is where the changes made become habits through continued practice and growth. Typical actions for family members include attending support group meetings, having a sponsor, sponsoring others, having appointments as needed, going to and helping with activities, and enhancing their relationship with their Higher Power. They are enforcing boundaries with love and not anger. They are letting go and letting God with love. It is common for a family member to stop having appointments during this phase. It is not unusual for a family member in the maintenance phase of recovery to leave the program. For the loved one, leaving recovery is unhealthy and usually leads to a severe relapse. This is not necessarily the case for the family member.

CODEPENDENT RECYCLE OR RELAPSE

Like substance users in recovery, codependents in recovery can relapse back into codependent behaviors. A codependent relapse initiates the overwhelming desire to rescue the loved one, punish the loved one, enable the loved one, or withdraw. Withdrawing includes withdrawing from recovery, family, and friends. External signs of a codependency relapse include not enforcing a boundary, increased anxiety, depression, giving into manipulation, giving into catastrophizing, or rescuing the loved one. Completely reverting to old behaviors is less common, but it does occur, especially after a loved one relapses. In this case, the family member may need to restart the recovery process from the beginning. Here are some suggestions for dealing with a relapse:

- **NORMALIZE CODEPENDENT RELAPSE.** In discussions about codependency, let them know that codependents relapse just like those with SUD. Like SUD relapse, codependent relapses can occur at any stage of recovery. Like the loved one after the loved one's relapse, ask them to focus on just doing the next right thing.

- **DEVELOP RELAPSE PREVENTION AND RESPONSE PLANS.** Like SUD relapse, a codependent relapse starts well before the actual relapse occurs. Like SUD relapse, the codependent relapse follows the same general path. The prevention and response plans allow the client to identify the warning signs of a relapse and then identify the steps needed to prevent or recover from the relapse. Chapter 8, Family Member Recovery Plan, has more information on developing relapse prevention and relapse-response plans.

- **CONFRONT THEM.** Sometimes, the family member is not aware they are relapsing. They misinterpret the relapse as a worsening of their situation or recovery is not working. It is helpful at this time to let them know that this is just a relapse and then remind them of the tools they can use to get out of the relapse.

- **REEXAMINE OR START THEIR RECOVERY PLAN.** Codependent relapses usually occur because the family member has stopped doing one or more recovery behaviors. Reviewing their recovery plan is an effective way to let the family member identify and disclose the parts of the plan they are no longer doing. If the family member does not have a recovery plan, encourage them to start developing one.

- **SHOW ACCEPTANCE AND UNCONDITIONAL LOVE.** We are including a reminder to be accepting and loving here because, after a codependent relapse, the family member is in a bad place and needs acceptance of who they are and where they are in the moment.

PARTING THOUGHTS ON THE STAGES OF CHANGE

Each person moves through the stages of change at their own pace. Regardless of the stage of change, instilling hope in a family member is always essential. Hope comes from meetings, sponsors, and the recovery coach. A practical method to restore hope in a family member is recalling their past successes. Dwelling on their successes when they occur reinforces the success. It supports the positive feelings that result from the family member doing the right thing, even if the right thing generates sadness and fear.

Not surprisingly, family members seeking help are usually ready to move into the preparation phase because things have become unbearable. This may not be the case for family members ordered to attend support group meetings by the courts or, in some cases, by their loved one's school. Family members forced to attend will often wait in the parking lot during the meeting or drop their loved one off and leave. They can be very resistant to the recovery process. It is important to remember that both categories of family members are usually hurting because of their loved one's illegal substance use or because of the consequences of their loved one's substance use. Family members often feel that they are being punished for their loved one's mistakes. If they are in Stage 1 or Stage 2 codependency, they believe, with some justification, that they do not need help. What they are doing is working for them and the rest of the family. Regardless of their codependency stage, moving from precontemplation to contemplation requires the family member to recognize and accept that they have a problem.

For some family members, as the loved one gets better, they begin to feel worse. As one mom put it, "My daughter was sober, my son was sober, my family was getting better, but it seemed like I felt worse." This is more common than expected and is not necessarily a relapse. There are several reasons why family members feel worse. First, the loved one's sobriety changes the family dynamics. During active SUD, the loved one was the family's focus, and family members were able to put aside other issues like their own substance use, their physical and mental health, their happiness, and their relationships with other family members. Now that the loved one is sober, family members can no longer avoid these issues.

Second, the SUD crisis can unmask past trauma or force repressed memories to the surface. A mother's memory of childhood abuse gradually surfaced during the family SUD crisis, along with severe post-traumatic stress disorder (PTSD). Her husband and counselor knew what was happening before she did. Both gently encouraged the mom to seek appropriate help. Eventually, the mom got the help she needed. Joanne Daxon's book, *A New Normal Now*, illustrates how this can happen (D. 2007).

Third, family members, especially parents/guardians, need to grieve what they lost because of their loved one's SUD. Chapter 16. Recognizing and Dealing with Grief addresses this topic in detail.

Actions for the recovery coach to consider when a loved one's sobriety makes a family member feel worse include:

- **NORMALIZE FAMILY MEMBERS FEELING WORSE WHEN THEIR LOVED ONE GETS BETTER.** A family member's life getting worse when a loved one is sober is counterintuitive and contrary to the narrative in most families: "If he would stop using, we would be fine." Let the family members know that this is a normal part of recovery.

- **RECOMMEND INDIVIDUAL THERAPY IF NEEDED.** Family members with mental disorders will need mental health specialists. This is especially true if the client is dealing with trauma. Be exceptionally watchful for the emergence of suppressed trauma during the recovery process.

- **RECOMMEND FAMILY OR MARRIAGE/COUPLES COUNSELING IF NEEDED.** One of the premises of our program is that individual recovery fosters family recovery. The dynamics of a family or a relationship may be such that the family needs specialized family or relationship counseling.

PART II

The Family Recovery Program

The family recovery program used in this book, is based on the integrated APG approach for family member recovery. Chapter 4, Integrated Alternative Peer Groups for Family Member Recovery, discusses the use of integrated APGs for family member recovery. It is important to remember that PDAP was a real grassroots organization built from the ground up. Like similar organizations, PDAP has undergone multiple transformations that led to PDAP becoming completely decentralized. As this decentralization occurred, many other organizations adopted and modified the PDAP approach. The approach presented in Chapter 4 is the approach the authors experienced in the PDAP organizations they attended and were later employed by.

CHAPTER 5, Integrated Alternative Peer Group Recovery Culture, discusses the recovery culture that is common to PDAP integrated APG-based organizations. All authors agree that culture is the "secret sauce" of the integrated APG approach. Chapter 5 does a deep dive into what the authors are calling the integrated APG culture with sufficient detail so you can incorporate the culture into your practice. It is important to remember that the decentralized nature of PDAP means each organization may or may not agree with what we have written.

CHAPTER 6, Family Group Meetings, describes the family meetings used by the authors. This description includes the purpose of each meeting and how to run them. Some of these meetings may not be appropriate for your organization or practice.

CHAPTER 7, Peer Coaching/Counseling Appointments, guides conducting appointments based on the author's approach to recovery. This includes actions the peer coach should take before the appointment, the conduct of the initial appointment, and follow-up appointments.

CHAPTER 8, Family Member Recovery Plan, provides a process to develop a holistic family member recovery plan. The four-step planning process includes identifying the family member's needs first and then identifying the family member's assets to address those needs. The third and fourth steps are goal identification and setting the objectives needed to attain the family member's goals.

CHAPTER 4

Integrated Alternative Peer Groups for Family Member Recovery

AA is the most famous peer group dedicated to helping people recover from SUD. Bill W. and Dr. Bob S., the founders of AA, designated June 10, 1935, as the start of AA because it was Dr. Bob S.'s sobriety date (Al-Anon Family Groups 2011). Al-Anon, a peer group for family members, had its beginning when Bill W. and Dr. Bob S.'s wives, Lois and Annie, respectively, met in June 1935 (Al-Anon Family Groups 2011). Like Bill W. and Dr. Bob S., Lois and Annie found that they could help each other deal with the alcoholism in their families. As AA meetings grew in size, the number of spouses in Lois and Annie's meetings also grew. As AA spread, so did these family member meetings. These family meetings became so widespread that in March 1945, the Alcoholic Foundation (forerunner to AA) officially recognized the family group APG, dubbed the Non-Alcoholic Family Group (Al-Anon Family Groups 2011). From then on, this family peer group rapidly grew and became the Al-Anon we know today.

Like AA and Al-Anon, Alateen was a grassroots organization. Teens were welcome at Al-Anon meetings, but many found they could not relate to the issues of the adult Al-Anon members. In addition, it was difficult for a teen to be completely open with a parent or other adult family member in the room. The book *Many Voices, One Journey* noted that teen-only meetings started as early as 1956, and Alateen was officially formed in 1957 (Al-Anon Family Groups 2011).

The gap in these groups was a specific group for teens and young adults with SUD. There are two reasons for this. First, alcoholism was, and, to a great extent, still is, a disease that afflicts older people. Second, when these groups were formed, teen substance use was not a significant issue. The widespread use of marijuana in the 60s and 70s changed this, and substance use became an issue for the young (Meehan, Beyond the Yellow Brick Road: Our Children and Drugs, Revised 2007). PDAP was another grassroots organization that filled this gap by establishing what came to be known as an integrated APG for teen substance users and a separate integrated APG for their families (PDAP 1982, PDAP 1990, Meehan, Beyond the Yellow Brick Road: Our Children and Drugs, Revised 2007, Cates and Cummings 2003).

Like AA, PDAP, the first integrated APG, started with the meeting of two people. The first was Bob Meehan, who was an alcoholic and heroin addict. The second was Father Charles Wyatt-Brown, the rector of the Palmer Episcopal Church in Houston, TX. Father Charlie gave Bob two jobs: the church janitor and talking to teens struggling with drug and alcohol use. Bob connected with teenagers because he was basically a teenager himself and showed them unconditional love, unconditional acceptance, and how to have sober fun. These became the three pillars of PDAP's teen APGs (Meehan, Beyond the Yellow Brick Road: Our Children and Drugs, Revised 2007). The first meeting of what became PDAP occurred in July 1971 and had six teenagers in attendance (PDAP 1982).

The PDAP Family Group, originally called the Parent Group, also started with people meeting each other. The parents who brought their teens to the meetings started "meeting around the coffee pot," and they found help and comfort in being together (PDAP 1982, PDAP 1990). Bob Meehan's wife, Joy, spearheaded adding the Parent Group to PDAP's structure. Through the years, the Parent Group changed its name to the Family Group because, like Al-Anon, PDAP recognized that the whole family needed help. (PDAP 1982, PDAP 1990)

This section will briefly summarize the integrated APG and how it is applied to family members. The books *Recovering Our Children: A Handbook for Parents of Young People in Early Recovery* by John C. Cates and Jennifer Cumming and the book *Beyond the Yellow Brick Road: Our Children and Drugs, Revised* by Bob Meehan provide detailed descriptions of the integrated APG approach to recovery (Cates and Cummings 2003, Meehan, Beyond the Yellow Brick Road: Our Children and Drugs, Revised 2007).

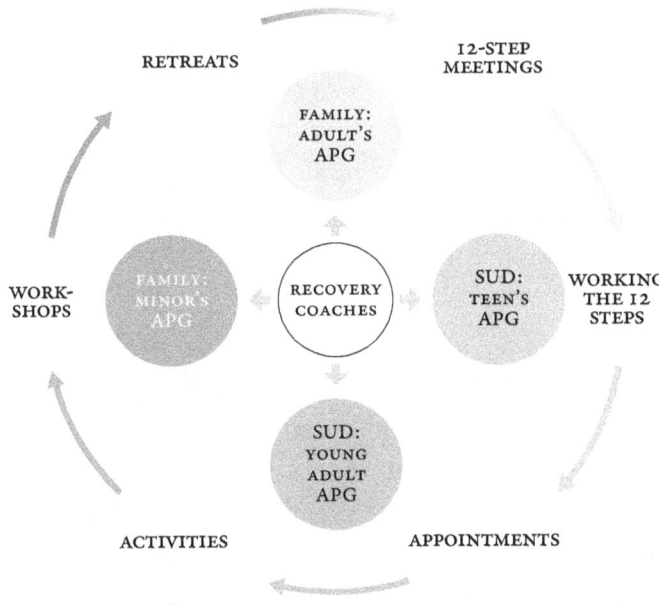

FIGURE 4. INTEGRATED ALTERNATIVE PEER
GROUP STRUCTURE AND PROCESSES

Figure 4 shows the basic structure of an integrated APG. Like AA, Al-Anon, and Alateen, the integrated APG is a peer-based recovery approach using the 12 Step process, which includes working the 12 Steps with a sponsor and attending 12 Step meetings. The first difference between an integrated APG and AA-type meeting is the organization has all groups under one umbrella. A typical integrated APG will have a teen group (typically 12 to 17 years old), a young adult group (typically 18 to 35 years old), a family group for adult family members (18 years old and older), and a family group for minors (typically 9 to 17 years old).[10]

The second difference is the presence of recovery coaches or counselors. Bob Meehan was the first recovery coach for the teens in PDAP. Bob had no formal training, but he had what has become the main qualification for integrated APG recovery coaches—lived experience. Bob knew what it was like to be dependent on substances as a teen. He was their peer. Similarly, Bob Meehan's wife, Joy, was the first family group coach. Similarly, she had no training, but she had the main qualification: she had lived experience as a family member (PDAP 1982). Recovery coaches guide meetings and coach/counsel group members. They also organize and run activities, workshops, and retreats. The advantage of having all groups in one organization is the staff's ability to discuss each family member to get a clear picture of what is happening in the family as a whole.

PARTING THOUGHTS ON THE INTEGRATED APG

There are multiple variations to the integrated APG described in this section. Sometimes, this approach is labeled enthusiastic recovery (Meehan, Beyond the Yellow Brick Road: Our Children and Drugs, Revised 2007), but there are commonalities. The first is the emphasis on having fun. As Bob Meehan put it, "The secret [to the program] is in showing adolescents that they can have fun without drugs and alcohol. And I mean "teen" fun not "adult" fun" (Meehan, Beyond the Yellow Brick Road: Our Children and Drugs, Revised 2007). The same is true for the family member. Having fun is a major driver for a family member to do the work needed for their recovery.

---

10 Chapter 6 has a more detailed discussion of the types and structure of these meetings.

CHAPTER 5

Integrated Alternative Peer Group Recovery Culture

A ll of the authors recovered in and worked for programs that used a PDAP-styled integrated APG approach to recovery for both persons with SUD and their families. All of the authors agree that these programs were so effective because of their culture. The purpose of this chapter is to describe the culture in sufficient detail to allow you to incorporate the culture into your work with family members. Specific objectives of this chapter include:

- Providing both an intellectual and an emotional understanding of each of the components of this culture.

- Providing specific guidance for using the concepts presented to help family members.

Figure 5, on the next page, has the key components of this recovery culture. Having fun is the basis of this culture because the program's primary focus was to help teens with SUD. Fun was a way to get teens to come and stay in the group. The founders of PDAP quickly found that fun was also crucial for family members. Like their loved ones, family members lost the ability to have fun. For family members, having fun helps them get their lives back and provides periods where their sole focus is not on their loved one. Like all 12-Step programs, God is at the center of recovery. God holds the other components together and provides the ability to accomplish each aspect of this culture.

As with many concepts, this culture has an intangible quality that a family member needs to experience to understand. We will use a drum circle analogy to share this culture's intangible aspects. Before getting into the drum circle, we must address the concept of God in a 12-Step program and God as a central part of our culture.

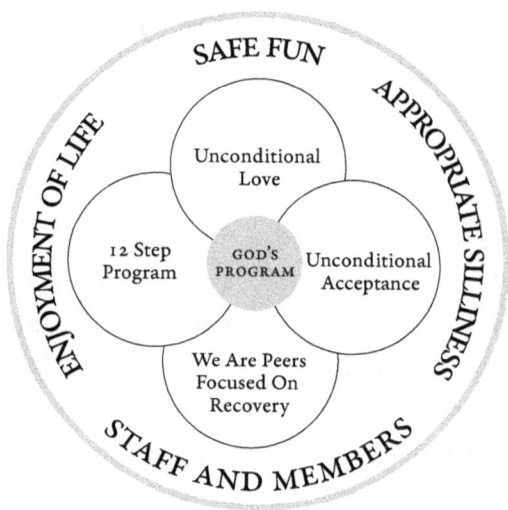

FIGURE 5. THE COMPONENTS OF THE RECOVERY CULTURE

A Higher Power We Have Chosen to Call God

As shown in *Figure 5*, God is central to the recovery culture. At first glance, this appears to be at odds with 12-Step recovery being non-sectarian. It is not at odds because of how 12-Step recovery programs incorporate God. In 12-Step cultures, God is not defined by a specific religion or limited by the organization. Each individual defines their Higher Power as a part of their recovery journey. The term often used is a God of our understanding. Some cite the concept of God or even the use of the word God as a significant obstacle to accepting the recovery culture. In many ways, the spiritual aspects of the 12 Steps are for people with these doubts and fears. In some cases, just the word "God" will cause some to reject this program. In these cases, we are kind to them and help them seek recovery elsewhere while praying that they gain the willingness to begin the spiritual journey of the 12 Steps. This journey ends with understanding God and accepting the word "God" without reservation.

Drum Circle: An Emotional Understanding

Imagine yourself in a drum circle with a group of people using percussion instruments. A leader sets the beat—thump, thump, thump—and another person controls the volume by raising or lowering their instrument.

Now, others choose to chime in one at a time, including you, all with their own distinct rhythm, but always in time with the beat set and at the same volume, getting louder and softer together. Once everyone is drumming, the circle and sound take on a life of its own, and there is an inexplicable feeling of community and connection.

Can you hear it? Good.

Imagine you hear someone in the circle trying to change the beat. It is tempting to choose to follow along, but the power of the circle keeps you and everyone else drumming to the original beat. Eventually, the person who went off course cannot help but fall back into the group's cadence. In another instance, someone other than the designated volume-control drummer wants to take over and determine how loud everyone plays. However, no one follows along. Again, in this instance, that person succumbs to the strength of the collective circle.

Why is this important? In each example, no one in the circle chose to ostracize, reprimand, or otherwise correct those participants who strayed. When the strays decided to return to the circle, the group welcomed them back without question or comment.

Now, we want you to think about two more drum circle scenarios. In one, a participant has a rhythm that annoys you. It is not just their rhythm but the instrument they are using. The sound is not pleasant to you in any way. In a normal situation, you would remove yourself so you would not have to hear something that grates your nerves. However, you have committed to this drum circle, so you stay. Moreover, you are glad you did. To your surprise, the sound was not annoying when that person joined the collective circle and aligned with the group's beat. It enriched the overall sound and the experience.

Finally, think about this. You are in a large drum circle, including at least 20 people choosing to participate. The beat and all the beautiful rhythms are loud and in full swing. One by one, the circle leader instructs the participants to stop drumming and fill a vial with sand. Surprisingly, when just one person among many stopped drumming, you noticed. You miss their rhythm. There is a hole in the sound, but the drum circle continues without disruption or missing a beat. Moreover, when that person rejoins the circle, their sound instantly fills the hole and is more appreciated and beautiful than if they had never stopped drumming.

It Is God's Program

THE BASIC BEAT

Central to any 12-Step program is turning our will and lives over to "...the care of God as we understand Him." This belief permeates every aspect of the culture. We are not in charge of our program. Our Higher Power is in charge. God's basic beat is what holds this program together. It allows people with vastly different rhythms to develop a space where others can seamlessly add their rhythms without condemnation or the requirement to change their rhythms.

Individual rhythms do change, but it is not the group that changes the rhythm; it is God. The group gives the members a safe place to open themselves to hear, feel, and sense God's basic beat. Hearing God's beat will either confirm your life's rhythm or reveal the rhythm you were born to have. Our Higher Power's beat and the group provide a safe place for the members to transform their rhythms.

Part of the recovery culture is the staff's commitment to working their 12-Step recovery program; as the 11th Step states, "To improve our conscious contact with our Higher Power, we have chosen to call God." The culture asks each staff member to commit to strengthening their understanding of God's beat in their lives and then changing the rhythm of their lives to align with their Higher Power's plan for them.

Enjoyment, Fun, Silliness

GOD'S JOY

Among other things, the drum circle is fun. That is why people stay in the circle and why they come back. Learning to have fun again and having fun is a crucial component of building the relationships needed for recovery for both the loved one and the family. The coaches and counselors have fun with each other and with the participants. It is often loud, sometimes obnoxious, silly fun that can, for instance, involve people singing joyfully off-key, playing baseball in the office, having office chair races, or filling offices with junk.

God's joy can involve high school students and coaches singing and playing so loud that there are complaints from the floors above and below. It can include teens wrapping a counselor like a Christmas present and then attempting to do a form of tap dance to put on social media. It often involves ropes courses, movie nights, sober parties, indoor rock climbing, sober proms, trips to the beach, fishing trips, camping (or glamping), or hiking. Contrary to what other organizations may think, the time spent in these activities is not wasted. This is time valuably spent in building the kind of spirituality and resilience that "sticks to the ribs." Family members and loved ones need this kind of spirituality and resilience to make it through another relapse or another crisis in the family. This is opening up to another individual in a very vulnerable way—letting someone inside where our Higher Power is. This embodies the promise, "We will know a new freedom and a new happiness."

The therapeutic value of fun for teens is teaching them that they can have fun without using mind-altering substances. It also gives them "war stories" to counter the stories their friends have about using substances. For example, one teen activity involved taking Nerf guns into a nearby hospital parking lot and playing war games. Someone in the hospital thought it was an active shooter and called a SWAT team. This is an extreme, hopefully not-to-be-repeated example of sober teens having a "war story" that would be hard to top.

Fun for family members is just as important because family members slowly forget how to have fun. Eric and Joanne recounted going on a drive to an amusement park after being in recovery for six months. Eric told a joke, and they laughed until they were in tears. They both looked at each other and said, "Wow! It has been a long time since we really laughed." For Eric and Joanne, it was almost a year and a half since they had laughed like that. Fun also fosters the relationships family members need in recovery.

Unconditional Love

UNCONDITIONAL LOVE IS A CONSCIOUS DECISION

Unconditional love for our clients, staff, and the people we encounter is vital to this culture. The closest description of this type of love is that it is an agape love. This extraordinary love is based on loving someone simply because you hear God's beat in them. It is like the decision to join the drum circle. The decision to overcome your hesitancy and start your rhythm in line with God's beat. The decision to accept the other members of the drum circle when they strayed, when they left, and when they returned.

Agape love is not romantic love; romantic love is part biochemical and part compatibility. It is not the love a parent has for a child. Familial love is part biochemical and part innate. It is not a love that you have for a close friend. Friendship-love grows because of similar interests, compatible personalities, and time spent together. Agape is a love that occurs because we choose to love the person without foreknowledge, attraction, or time spent together. We choose to love the person as soon as they walk through the door. We choose to love because our Higher Power does not make junk. We choose to love because each of us has felt the power of agape love.

DIFFERENT TYPES OF LOVE

The English language has only one word for love, which includes a range of emotions from erotic love to agape love. Understanding each distinct type of love is essential to fully understanding the unconditional agape love that is a part of our culture. *Table 2* on the next page has the seven types of love in the Greek language.

TABLE 2. TYPES OF LOVE (PAULCHAPMAN.COM 2019,
STEPS OF FAITH 2020, M. G. WHITE N.D.)

Type of Love	Definition
Eros	Deep physical attraction to another that includes passion, lust, and intense sexual desire.
Agape	It is choosing to love someone simply because of their humanity—a selfless, sacrificial love.
Philia	Affectionate love like the love between good friends that does not include sexual desire. This is brotherly love.
Storge	The love that family members have for one another is mainly used to describe the love between a parent and child.
Pragma	Enduring love. This is the love from long-term relationships where there is a deep commitment.
Philautia	Self-love or self-compassion. This refers to healthy self-esteem, which impacts how we treat and interact with others and enables us to give and accept love.
Ludas	Playful love, like flirting or having a crush on someone. This often happens at the beginning of a relationship that may or may not last.

The group and the culture are built on fostering pragma, storge, philia, philautia, and especially agape. In the drum circle analogy, agape love provides the ability to join the drum circle. No one in the circle knows your rhythm. No one knows if they will like your rhythm, but God's beat in you and the drum circle creates acceptance. Once you add your rhythm, you notice how your rhythm enriches the drum circle. This is philautia. The group welcomes you into the circle. You are worthy of being in the circle. As the beat continues, a feeling of connection starts to grow, and you feel a bond with those around you, and that bond grows to philia. You begin to feel a special connection with some rhythms that grow into a family-like bond—storge. As the drum circle continues, storge can grow into an enduring love or pragma. Agape, philautia, philia, storge, and pragma are the bedrock of healthy groups that provide the emotional and spiritual support needed by all in the group.

Without exception, expressions of eros and ludas are prohibited at meetings, activities, coaching/counseling sessions, or between sponsors and sponsees. Ludas and eros have a wonderful place in committed relationships. Still, ludas and especially eros significantly hinder the development of agape, philia, storge, pragma, and philautia because they are, by our Higher Power's design, self-centered and selfish forms of love. Unfortunately, today's culture equates all forms of love to eros. This leads to the misconception that eros is a component of each of the other forms of love.

FORGIVENESS

Agape love is the cornerstone of the 12-Step process that allows the performance of one of the most challenging tasks—forgiving someone you do not like or even may despise. Deciding to see the humanity in that person, deciding to see God's spark, choosing to see His love for that person, choosing to feel our Higher Power's beat in that person; all these are required to break down the walls of bitterness and hate and allow real forgiveness to occur. Real forgiveness is what rids a person of resentment. This is why experiencing agape love is vital to the recovery process. It is not easy to give or accept if agape love is not known or experienced.

Forgiving someone that hurt you does not mean you will like them; it does not mean you will not hold them accountable or enter a relationship with them. It does mean that they will no longer be in control of part of your life. A recovery saying illustrates the impact of holding on to resentment. "Holding on to a resentment is like drinking poison and expecting the other person to die."

KIND VS. NICE

> "When I was nice, I was taking care of my daughter. When I was kind, God was taking care of my daughter." Debi, a Family Group member

Our unconditional love is a "kind" love, not a "nice" love. Kind and nice are closely related words that many believe are quite different, and the difference is essential in recovery (Blackburn Center 2020, Caparrotta 2020, Shi 2016). "Nice" is often described as being pleasing or agreeable, while "kind" is often described as acting out of a sense of benevolence and caring. Putting it more plainly, nice is giving someone what they want. It is giving a child all the candy they want. Nice is not taking the child to the dentist because the child is afraid. Nice is paying bail for someone arrested on drug charges. Nice is paying the rent and providing food for a needy family member with SUD.

Kind is giving someone what they need, whether they want it or not. Kind is regulating the candy intake of a child and taking them to the dentist. The dentist can cause pain but does not harm the child. Going to the dentist benefits the child in the long run. Kind is letting the loved one with SUD feel the consequences of their drug use. Kind is not bailing someone out, not paying the rent, and not buying food. Kind is calling the police when that is the right thing to do. Kind is not allowing them to take advantage of you. Kind is not wanting their recovery more than they do. Kind is recognizing that you are just as important as they are. Kind is enforcing a tough boundary. These acts of kindness can be painful for the loved one and the family member, but they are what the loved one needs for their sobriety. They are also what family members need for their recovery.

In the drum circle, when someone chooses to move away from our beat, kind is not moving with them to make them feel better. We maintain the beat so that they may feel the absence of our Higher Power in their lives. It is an unsettling feeling to break away and be alone. This loneliness is the feeling that can eventually bring them back to the circle. Kindness is letting them feel the loneliness separation from God causes. Nice would be comforting them in their loneliness so they never feel the need to return to God.

UNCONDITIONAL LOVE: NOT UNCONDITIONAL "LIKE" NOR UNCONDITIONAL "TRUST"

Agape love does not require that you like the person, nor does it require that you trust the person. You can dislike a person but still choose to love them. You can distrust a person but still choose to love them. This is analogous to choosing to love someone whose individual rhythm is not one to your liking by loving the beat of our Higher Power within them,

It is important to remember that trust has two components. The first is honesty. Does the person mean what they are saying? The second is ability. Do they have the ability to do what they are saying they will do? A loved one not in recovery might say, "This is the last time I will ever use." They might mean this with all their heart, so they are being honest. They are not trustworthy, however, because, more than likely, they do not have the tools (the ability) to stay sober. Not trusting an untrustworthy person is the kindest thing you can do for yourself and them.

UNCONDITIONAL ACCEPTANCE

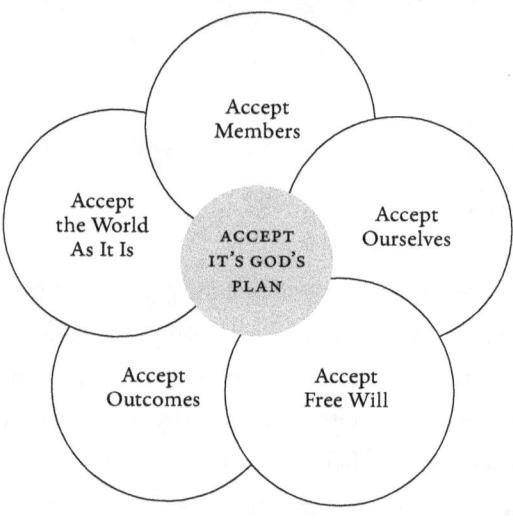

FIGURE 6. UNCONDITIONAL ACCEPTANCE

Figure 6 above illustrates the six aspects of our unconditional acceptance. We unconditionally accept our members, ourselves, everyone's free will, outcomes, and the world as it is. We accept that God's plan and not our plan matters. The drum circle analogy illustrates aspects of unconditional acceptance. Each member freely chooses to join the drum circle and comes to the circle with their rhythm. We accept their rhythm. We do not ask them to meet us where we are, but we meet them where they are. Anyone can join our drum circle, and the circle will welcome them.[11] Our only requirement is a willingness to enter recovery. If they are in a meeting, attending an activity, or an appointment, whether they will admit it or not, they have a willingness to recover.

---

11 They can join if they do not jeopardize the safety of the people in the group. Most PDAP-like groups have three rules to keep our members safe—the three F's - for our meetings and activities. There is no "fixing"—being high or in possession. There is no fighting. There is no "flirting"—having sex or trying to pick up people. These rules are in place to protect members from the most common forms of abuse—drug abuse, physical abuse, and sexual abuse.

WE ACCEPT OUR HIGHER POWER'S PLAN

Acceptance of our Higher Power's plan is the basic beat of the culture and what drives unconditional acceptance in the program. We accept that God can fundamentally change people because God has fundamentally changed us, and we have witnessed fundamental changes in our members. The basic beat of God's plan brought order, fellowship, acceptance, purpose, and contentment to our chaotic lives. These changes sometimes happen quickly and sometimes occur slowly.

We also accept that we do not and cannot understand our Higher Power's plan for us, nor can we know why He ordained our path or our members' paths. Each member has a different rhythm, different gifts, and different weaknesses. We may not understand the rhythm of a person's life. We may not like the rhythm of a person's life. We know that the rhythm is our Higher Power's rhythm for that person. We accept that we may never know why God gave them that rhythm.

We accept that this program is not our program but our Higher Power's program. We acknowledge that we do not cause change in our members. God's beat causes the change. Recovery is not about us. Recovery is about our Higher Power. Sometimes, we correctly observe that our Higher Power is not nice. He often refuses to give us what we want. Sometimes, the work we need to do is painful. In all

> **SELF ACCEPTANCE**
>
> "I always thought I was selfless, and humble. I worked with a therapist for a while and at the right moment, the therapist said, 'I need to tell you that you are very self-centered.' I was stunned and angry. Around the same time my sponsor told me that I was a very prideful person. I was stunned and angry again. In rebuttal, I told my sponsor that, 'I was the humblest person I know.' (I believe my objection proved my sponsor's case.) These good men allowed me to see reality. I now know I was a prideful, self-centered person.
>
> Instead of beating myself up, I felt relieved because now everything made sense. I accepted that I was a selfish, prideful person. Knowing what I really needed to work on, I work on it. Real growth occurred and real recovery occurred because I accepted myself as I was and not as I thought I was. Seeing and accepting reality relieved and refreshed me."
>
> FAMILY GROUP MEMBER

instances, our Higher Power is kind. He gives us what we need. This applies to our recovery. It also applies to our members' recovery.

WE ACCEPT OUR MEMBERS

> "We accept people where they are and meet them where they are. We have to because where else could they be but where they are?" Anonymous

We unconditionally accept a person with SUD or a family member as a member of our program and someone deserving of our love and acceptance. We recognize that God's basic beat is in each one of us. Our knowledge of our Higher Power's beat in us and our lives allows us to sense and accept those most would consider unacceptable.

Unconditional acceptance does not mean approval of a member's actions or lifestyle. We unconditionally accept the substance user, but we disapprove of substance use. We unconditionally accept a member who has committed a crime, but we disapprove of the crime. We unconditionally accept a parent who is enabling their loved one, but we disapprove of enabling. We disapprove of a parent not setting and enforcing boundaries, but we will accept and love that parent.

Unconditional acceptance is meeting people where they are, not where we think they should be. We do not ask them to move towards us. We move toward them. Standing where they stand, we share our experience, love, and understanding. Sobriety from substances and codependency is our goal, but we do not require sobriety for acceptance, but rather a willingness to be sober.

Unconditional acceptance does not mean we will change our core beliefs or culture if they are at odds with a potential member's beliefs. Here are some specific examples of core beliefs:

- **WE ARE A PEER-BASED PROGRAM.** Our program is for people who are dealing with a loved one abusing substances. We will help people dealing with other issues find appropriate help.

- **WE ARE A 12-STEP PROGRAM.** Many do not believe in 12-Step programs. We will not change our 12-Step approach but guide the person to alternative resources.

- **WE ARE A GOD-BASED PROGRAM.** Atheists, agnostics, and those who have a dread of God or the word God are welcome in our program. They may choose not to join or to leave, but they are welcome.

WE ACCEPT OURSELVES

Unconditionally accepting our members requires unconditional acceptance of ourselves as we are in the moment. This self-acceptance implies understanding the need to work through denial and self-deception to reveal all our warts and halos—weaknesses and strengths. Once we see the character defects (e.g., false pride, selfishness), the character strengths (honesty, willingness), the wrongs against us, and the wrongs we committed, we decide to accept ourselves because this is who our Higher Power made us to be in this moment. This acceptance allows real change to occur because we can see our reality. We model this for our clients and provide them with the tools to make their recovery journey.

WE ACCEPT THAT ALL, INCLUDING OUR LOVED ONES, HAVE FREE WILL

The three C's are commonly used in recovery circles: "You did not cause it (SUD). You cannot cure it. You cannot control it." At the heart of a good deal of a family member's misery is believing the opposite. The family member, especially a parent or guardian, believes they did cause it, can control it, and can cure it. Family members, friends, and pastors often reinforce this belief by telling the family members directly or indirectly that it is their fault. Giving a family member unsolicited advice is an indirect way of telling a family member that the loved one's SUD is their fault. "You need to give her goals." "You need to come down hard on him." This "advice" implies the parent did not do these things or did not know they were supposed to do them. The loved one will add to the chorus by also blaming the parents.

A family member's peers, friends, and pastors sometimes fail to consider that our Higher Power has granted us all free will, and we all, including our loved ones, have the power of choice. All SUD starts with a choice, the choice to use mind-altering substances for the first time. The choice is illegal for those under 21 years of age. First-use has multiple reasons: wanting acceptance, wanting to self-medicate, wanting to escape, or just wanting to feel good. Despite these reasons, first-use is still a choice.

WE ACCEPT OUTCOMES

When a drum circle starts, all we can control is our choice to join the drum circle and our rhythm. We cannot control the final sound of the drum circle because we do not control all the factors that contribute to it. For most family members, accepting outcomes is a difficult concept, which is why most will believe that they caused their loved one's addiction, they can cure it, and they can control it. Their loved ones, non-recovery friends, and non-recovery family members will reinforce these beliefs. Finally, outcomes are beyond our control because many things beyond our control determine outcomes. Our drumbeat, however, is something we can control.

The primary uncontrollable for family and friends is the decision-making of our loved ones. Our Higher Power gave us all free will. Despite the best training and mentoring, many make harmful choices. The second uncontrollable is genetics. A genetic component of SUD is beyond the control of parents and families. The third is the substance-induced changes in the biochemical processes in the brain. These are the changes that can lead to SUD.

A Peer-Based Program for the Whole Family

This book outlines a peer-based program for family members. The primary qualification for our coaches and counselors is that they are peers. The primary qualification for being in a drum circle is to have a percussion instrument. Family group counselors/coaches have been family members in a family dealing with SUD. Counselors/coaches for people with SUD are in recovery from SUD.

There are multiple specialties trained to work with people with SUD and their family members that do not require the counselor to be a peer. The bedrock of this approach is peers working with peers. There are two reasons for this. The first is the difference between sympathy and empathy. Sympathy is the ability to imagine or understand the feelings a person is having. Empathy is the ability to share someone's feelings because you have also experienced these feelings. This is the difference between thinking you understand what someone is going through and understanding what they are going through. This is the difference between looking at a picture of someone in a foxhole and being in the foxhole.

There is a second, more subtle reason for coaches working with family members to be peers—people who had loved ones with SUD. At some point in the recovery process, each viewed the other as the source of their misery. Even after working through resentments, both residual resentments and residual cultural biases remain, affecting the approach to recovery in casual conversations and more subtle ways. A good example is a sobriety T-shirt made by an organization. It had the following printed on it, "Sober AF." The AF stood for

"As F**k." A parent cringed at the cursing because of the cursing their loved one did when he/she used substances. The person recovering from SUD laughed. Coaches in recovery from SUD wanted the parents to change and to accept the language. Family coaches want the language to change because of how hurtful the language was to parents.

THIS IS A 12-STEP PROGRAM.

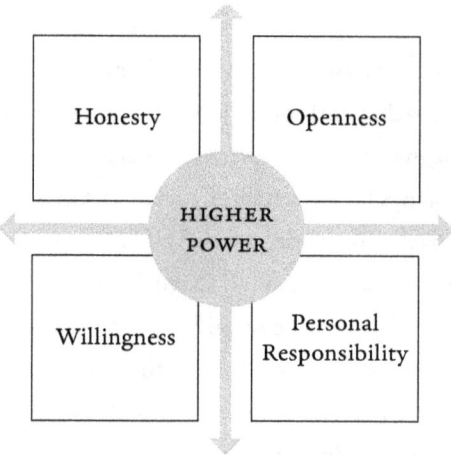

FIGURE 7. CORE VALUES OF A 12 STEP PROGRAM

This is a 12-Step program. *Table 3* on the next page shows the 12 Steps of AA (Alcoholics Anonymous 2019). For family members, the word "alcoholic" in Step 1 is replaced by the "loved one" who has SUD. In Step 2, it is SUD that causes the insanity in our loved ones. For family members, it is the obsessive, all-consuming focus on the loved one's disease. Five core values (*Figure 7*, above) are inherent in the 12 Steps—a Higher Power, honesty, openness, willingness, and personal responsibility.

TABLE 3. THE 12 STEPS OF AA

Step 1	We admitted we were powerless over alcohol—that our lives had become unmanageable.
Step 2	Came to believe that a Higher Power greater than ourselves could restore us to sanity.
Step 3	We made a decision to turn our will and our lives over to the care of God as we understand Him.
Step 4	Made a searching and fearless moral inventory.
Step 5	Admitted to God, to ourselves, and another human being the exact nature of our wrongs.
Step 6	Were entirely ready to have God remove all these defects of character.
Step 7	Humbly asked Him to remove our shortcomings.
Step 8	Made a list of all persons we had harmed and became willing to make amends to them all.
Step 9	Made direct amends to such people except when to do so would injure them or others.
Step 10	Continued to take personal inventory and when we were wrong promptly admitted it.
Step 11	Sought through prayer and meditation to improve our conscious contact with God as we understand Him, praying only for knowledge of his will for us and the power to carry that out.
Step 12	Having had a spiritual awakening as a result of these steps, we tried to carry this message to alcoholics, and to practice these principles in our affairs.

A HIGHER POWER

A belief in a Higher Power is central to all 12-Step programs. Except for admitting our powerlessness (Step 1.), each significant step in the process is preceded by work on our relationship with our Higher Power. The inventory (Step 4) is preceded by doing the work needed to believe that there is a power greater than us and that our Higher Power could restore us to sanity. This is a belief step, and it requires a decision to believe that there is a Higher Power, a benevolent power, who can restore us to sanity. This belief is a prerequisite to deciding to turn all that you are over to your Higher Power (Step 3.). These steps lay the groundwork for doing the inventory (Steps 4 and 5) that will relieve the resentments blocking the family member's recovery.

The relief a family member has after sharing their inventory can accomplish several important tasks. First, their relief strengthens their faith in the program. Second, they regain some of their ability to show love for their loved one. Third, the relief they feel strengthens their relationship with their Higher Power. Fourth, it facilitates the identification and removal of character defects. Character defects are often born, nurtured, and driven by resentments.

Steps 6 and 7 are essential for family members because they emphasize the importance of becoming willing to engage their Higher Power (Step 6) and the importance of humbling ourselves by asking God to remove our shortcomings. The subtle message in Step 7 is that we do not have the power to remove our shortcomings; only God has that ability. A family member must understand this subtle message because it can eliminate the frustration when a family member does the work, and their shortcomings remain.

A family member relayed the story of his jealousy. The jealousy of his wife's affection came into force when addiction hit his family. He did the work, did his inventory, made amends, and did it all again. The jealousy remained. One day, his wife said something that should have made him jealous. He was not jealous. This was so surprising that he started looking around, wondering where the jealousy went. From then on, he realized he had to do the work, and the defect would be gone when God was ready. God relieved him of the burden of removing his character defect. That was God's job. His job was to do the work.

The effect of the God-steps was to build a more trusting, more intimate relationship with the family member's Higher Power. This relationship enables a family member to do one of the hardest things they need to do—let go of their loved one and let God take care of him/her.

HONESTY

Rigorous personal honesty is a requirement for 12-Step programs and is also the bedrock of this culture. Rigorous honesty is like your rhythm in the drum circle. You enter the drum circle as the authentic you, and the drum circle accepts the authentic you. Recovery is partly about uncovering the authentic you, the "you" that your Higher Power is calling you to be. This process requires being honest with yourself and those around you. An anonymous member of a family group put it this way:

> When I first entered the program, despite all the evidence to the contrary, I believed I could manage my life. I knew it was unmanageable, but I refused to admit it. I was being dishonest. The first time I worked on Step 1, I realized my life was unmanageable. I believed that my life's unmanageability was due to my loved one's substance use, and I had no part in the unmanageability. If they would stop using drugs, my life would be manageable again.
>
> I was honest with myself and those around me because I believed that was the case. I did not have the recovery beliefs, the knowledge, or the understanding to recognize my part in my misery. As I learned about codependency and SUD and experienced group members getting their lives back even though their loved ones were still using, I came to believe that my life was unmanageable because of how I was responding to the SUD in my family. I was initially in denial about my part in my misery, but it was an honest denial. My genuine

acceptance of what I was learning and what the group was teaching allowed me to know and accept who I was at that moment—my authentic self.

The willingness to accept reality—being honest—in Steps 4 and 9 is an absolute requirement to remove the resentments and the guilt that are significant obstacles to becoming the natural, authentic person our Higher Power calls us to be.

OPENNESS

Openness is being open to recovery, the process, and the changes recovery brings. It is like being open enough to add your rhythm to the drum circle. Being open to the possibility that this new way of life could restore our sanity was the first step in openness. As the journey continues, we are open to whatever our Higher Power has in store for us. Openness starts with:

- Being open to having a relationship with a loving Higher Power. As recovery progresses, this changes to being open to having a more intimate relationship with God (Palmer Drug Abuse Program 1990).

- Being open to trusting the group and trusting the love of the group (Palmer Drug Abuse Program 1990). Trust that this agape love is real and that the people in the room care about you. Being open with other safe people allows us to speak our truth. It is also essential because it will enable us to feel the unconditional love and acceptance that is a part of the process. Being appropriately open with safe people is critical. A safe person will not exploit or hurt you because of your openness. A safe person is also someone whom your openness will not hurt. An example of hurting someone with openness is talking about your infidelities in a meeting where your spouse is present.

- Being open to forgiving people and making amends when required.

WILLINGNESS

Becoming willing to change is an often overlooked step in the change process. At this point, honesty has allowed the clear identification of character defects and how we have harmed others. The next step is gaining the willingness to change and then gaining the willingness to take the actions needed to enter recovery. Being open to change allows the person to identify the required changes, consider the actions they need, and imagine their lives after the changes. Just as importantly, being willing to change encourages accepting the support necessary to effect change in someone's life.

The 12-Step process asks for willingness to have our Higher Power remove our character defects and willingness to make amends to people we have harmed. Action steps follow each of these "willingness" steps. Step 6 is about becoming ready (or willing) to have God remove our character defects. After this comes Step 7, asking God to remove our character defects. Step 8 is becoming ready and willing to make amends to the people harmed. Then, Step 9 is making amends. The willingness steps are necessary because they acknowledge that many are not ready to forgive or make amends. Work on Steps 6 and 8 targets the barriers to willingness. Sometimes, the willingness to take the next step is a bridge too far for the family member. In these cases, the ask becomes working to become willing to be willing.

PERSONAL RESPONSIBILITY

We are only responsible for our rhythm, but we are 100% responsible for our rhythm. Our rhythm, the things we can control, includes what we say, do, think, believe, and feel. The first two—what we do and what we say—are obvious components of recovery. In Steps 8 and 9, we take responsibility for the hurtful things we said and did by making amends and offering restitution if possible. Steps 8 and 9 also require us to take responsibility for what we think, believe, and feel.[12] Our thoughts, our feelings, and our beliefs are precursors to the actions we take.[13] Steps 4 and 5 require us to take responsibility for our resentments because resentment is a feeling linked to a thought about a past, hurtful event.

Resentments are related to beliefs. Sometimes, a non-recovery belief caused resentment. For example, Eric Daxon resented his dad coming home drunk. When Eric thought about it as an adult, he was angry at the way his dad acted and the verbal fights his dad had with Eric's mom. Eric's anger was based on the belief that his dad could control his drinking. When Eric came to believe that SUD was a disease, his anger turned to sadness and compassion for the good man who had an awful disease. Eric was able to forgive his dad, and the resentment dissipated.

Application of the Culture

The purpose of this section is to guide the application of this culture to working with family members.

---

12   It is important to note that we are responsible for our feelings and not our emotions. An emotion is an immediate response to an event. Someone jumps out of a dark alley, and you immediately respond with fight, flight, or freeze. The difference between feelings and emotions is discussed further in Chapter 15, Moving from Non-recovery Beliefs to Recovery Beliefs.

13   How thoughts and feelings are precursors to action is discussed in more detail also in Chapter 15, Moving from Non-recovery Beliefs to Recovery Beliefs.

LEARN TO LIVE THE CULTURE

The first step in using this culture is learning to live the culture yourself. This is not as hard as it may seem because this is the culture for most 12-Step groups. There are sometimes unexpected obstacles. The most challenging concept for recovery coaches recovering from SUD is unconditional acceptance and unconditional love for the family member. The difficulty usually arises because they view the family member through the tinted lens of their codependent family.

Warning signs of this difficulty include telling degrading jokes or humorous stories about codependents, getting angry when a family member describes codependent behavior toward their loved one, and using unusually caustic language when talking to family members. Then there is the other extreme. A coach will take on the family member's pain. One coach said he returned to his office and cried after talking to family members. He was grieving what his disease put his parents through.

If you notice you are doing this, please do not ignore it. Family members can be hypersensitive to your affect, word choice, and body language. In cultural terms, these resentments are blocking your ability to provide the agape love needed to foster change in the family member. Work with your sponsor or a therapist to resolve these resentments.

INCORPORATING CULTURE INTO WORK WITH FAMILY MEMBERS

Each cultural concept is essential for the recovery of loved ones and the family. Full incorporation of these concepts by family members usually requires working the 12 Steps because of the pivotal role resentments and guilt play in blocking their full adoption. The coach can assist by introducing these concepts where appropriate in individual sessions and authentically sharing the culture's impact on their lives and recovery. The following are the most common family member roadblocks to accepting the culture and suggested methods to overcome these blocks.

- **THE MYTH THAT UNCONDITIONAL ACCEPTANCE MEANS GIVING UP.** It is common for a family member to struggle with acceptance because they believe acceptance means condoning their loved one's substance use and giving up. It is helpful to coach family members to approach acceptance from the perspective of needing to see things as they are so they can work on fixing the actual problem.

- **CONFUSING UNCONDITIONAL LOVE WITH UNCONDITIONAL TRUST AND UNCONDITIONAL LIKE.** Family members often conflate unconditional love with trust, liking someone, and being nice. One family member stated, "I believed if I loved my daughter, I had to trust and like her. I did not trust her or like her, so I thought I did not love her." What helps is pointing out that this is a program of unconditional love, not unconditional trust nor unconditional like. Trust is earned, and so is being liked. An anonymous parent stated, "This concept helps me because I did not like my loved one, and I did not trust my loved one. It was a relief to find I could love someone I did not trust or like."

- **KIND VS NICE.** Talking about allowing consequences and enforcing boundaries as being "kind" and enabling as being "nice" is a way of getting the point across in terms that are accurate and more palatable for the family member. Allowing the consequences and enforcing the boundaries is often called tough love. Reframing enforcing consequences and boundaries as kindness is accurate and meets the family where they are. They want to be kind to their loved ones.

The change in a family member's demeanor is striking when they understand that enforcing a boundary is one of the most loving and kind things they can do *for* their loved one. There is another benefit to framing boundaries as loving and kind. It fosters loving versus angry language when the family member talks to their loved one.

Parting Thoughts on the Culture

This recovery culture provides the structure to support each person's unique recovery journey. In the drum circle analogy, each person's unique instrument and rhythm symbolizes their journey. The drum circle provides the unconditional love and unconditional acceptance needed to ease the fear and anxiety of first joining the drum circle and second allowing the drum circle to hear their current rhythm. As the drum circle continues, the person hears the rhythm changes in other drum circle participants and watches the drum circle, not criticizing but accepting these personal changes. Much to the person's surprise, the circle accepts people failing, even leaving, and then welcomes them back. This accepting, loving "drum circle" gives the person the courage and support to seek, adopt, and internalize each of the 12 Steps' spiritual values.

CHAPTER 6

Family Group Meetings

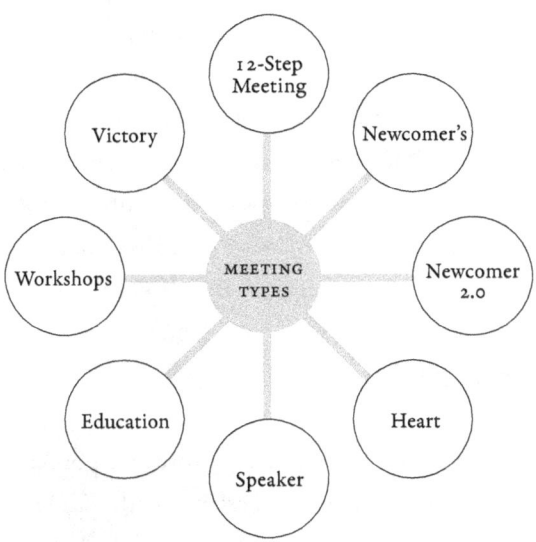

FIGURE 8. FAMILY GROUP MEETING TYPES
FOR PDAP-STYLE PROGRAMS

The meetings described in this section are based on the author's experiences in the primarily PDAP-styled programs they were associated with. *Figure 8* above shows the eight types of meetings common in a PDAP-styled family group.[14] These meetings have similar purposes: establishing group member connections,

---

14 The meetings shown in the figure are specific to the PDAP groups the authors were a part of. Other PDAP organizations may or may not include all of the meetings shown.

providing education, and supporting members in their recovery. Most 12-Step recovery programs have 12-Step meetings, newcomers' meetings, speaker meetings, education meetings, and workshops. Newcomers 2.0, heart meetings, and Victory Meetings are specific to some PDAP-styled organizations.

Adult Family Group 12-Step Meeting

Family Group 12-Step meetings are the foundation of the family program. In most respects, these support group meetings are like Al-Anon and Nar-anon meetings, except there are trained recovery coaches in the meetings. Specifically, these are support group meetings for adult family members (18 years old and older) dealing with SUD in their families. Family Group meetings provide affiliational support by providing a safe place for family members to share their stories, successes, and failures in recovery. It is also where a family member can form the deep personal connections that lead to finding a sponsor and wanting to participate in activities with other family members. A group meeting provides a safe venue for shared learning from people who are or have been in similar situations.

The recovery coaches have three and only three purposes in a family group 12-Step meeting: to share their own experience with SUD in their family, to keep the meeting safe, and to gain insights that may be helpful during coaching sessions. It is important to note that the coaches are neither moderators nor facilitators. They are just members of the group. Recovery coaches must remember that a group meeting is not a place for counseling individuals or giving them advice directly or indirectly.

Meetings are also a place for members to practice the principles of recovery in a safe environment. They are places where members can be honest, open, and willing without being judged. Members can learn to be accountable for their actions and experience the freedom that comes with this accountability. Practicing the principles of recovery in a meeting enhances the family member's ability to apply these principles in their daily lives.

Family members learn in a group meeting by listening to members share their experiences, love, and understanding. Each member is free to evaluate what group members are saying and decide if it will work for them without interference from anyone else. A common saying in the group is, "Take what you need and leave the rest." If members disagree with an approach, they are free not to use it.

PEER RECOVERY COACH SHARING THEIR EXPERIENCES

A peer coach sharing their experience, love, and understanding can be powerful for the group if the coach is sharing for the benefit of the group and not themselves. A family group meeting is not where a coach can work through their own issues. There are two reasons for a peer coach to share in a meeting. The first is to get the meeting back on track. Often, especially with newcomers, the sharing is not on topic; it has devolved into a member recounting their day, or the sharing includes collective pronouns and "you shoulds." If it makes the meeting unsafe, the peer coach needs to intervene directly. If not, the peer coach can redirect the meeting by sharing on the topic from the "I" perspective.

The second is injecting a recovery principle that the group, not individuals, needs to hear. If several members in the meeting struggle with a common concept, the peer coach can illustrate the recovery concept from their own experience. The most common is the "3 C's." A recovery coach sharing their struggles with the 3 C's, how they dealt with the battle, and where they are now will help the group grow. If an individual needs help, it is best to talk to that person after the meeting.

A peer coach sharing to break the silence is unacceptable. Silence in a meeting is often a good thing. It can provide the time needed for a member to find the words to express what they want to say. Silence gives the member who needs to share but is hesitating a little shove. Silence can also mean the group is just thinking. Eric has a story to remember when you want to "break the silence:" Eric was in an appointment with a woman who needed to share at a meeting. Eric knew that because she told him. She told Eric that someone jumped in whenever she was about to share. One person said they jumped in because they could not stand the silence. It is not encouraged but acceptable for a group member to break the silence. A peer coach sharing to break the silence is unacceptable and not encouraged.

The coach decides when continued silence no longer benefits the group. Rather than sharing to break the silence, the coach can end the meeting early by asking if anyone has a "burning desire." A burning desire is something a person needs to say before leaving the meeting, and it can be on any topic. Commonly, asking for burning desires prods a person into sharing something they wanted but could not bring themselves to share.

KEEPING A MEETING SAFE

The priority for coaches/counselors in a meeting is to keep the meeting safe for the participants. *Figure 9* below shows the components of a safe meeting. The following is a discussion of each of these elements:

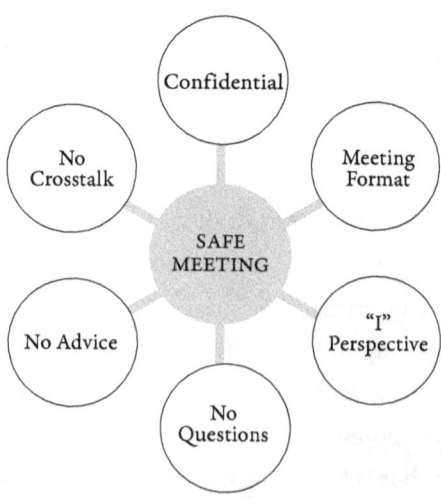

FIGURE 9. MEETING-SAFETY GUIDELINES

- **ENSURE THE MEETING REMAINS CONFIDENTIAL.** Confidentiality is the most crucial aspect of keeping meetings safe. What is said and who is in a meeting are confidential and not discussed with people not in the meeting. There are exceptions, and these include suspected child abuse or elder abuse or someone in the meeting who is considering suicide.[15] If the participants are virtual, they must be in a place where non-participants cannot see or hear the other people in the meeting.

  Actions that facilitate confidentiality include reminding members at the beginning of a meeting about confidentiality and its importance. Second, the peer coach can gently confront someone who is breaking confidentiality. Confronting when you become aware of someone breaking confidentiality is important because otherwise, you implicitly approve the breach.

- **MAINTAIN STANDARD MEETING FORMAT.** Formally opening and formally closing a meeting makes it clear when the meeting guidelines apply and when they do not. Asking people to say, "Hi, my name is..." when they want to share ensures everyone knows who has the floor to speak. Saying the first name also enhances the intimacy of the group. Learning people's names fosters intimacy and helps members get sponsors. Asking members to let the group know they finished sharing makes it clear that they have indeed finished sharing. This rule is important because sometimes a family member is silent because they

---

15 There are federal and state-specific requirements for reporting child abuse, elder abuse, and suicidal ideation. Most organizations have internal policies to implement or supplement federal and state requirements. Please ensure you are familiar with these.

are trying to find the words to say something very painful. With this rule in place, the group knows to wait.

The coach must maintain the same meeting format regardless of the group size. Group members, especially new members, find comfort and safety in knowing what will happen next in a meeting. As one coach said, "The meeting was small, and I suggested that we just talk instead of having a regular meeting. I sensed the tension in the room when I said that. One member started to walk out of the meeting." Some family members only attend support group meetings because the meeting format makes it safe for them.

- ENSURE GROUP MEMBERS SHARE FROM THE "I" PERSPECTIVE. We primarily ask members to share from the "I" perspective *to keep the meeting safe*. When the person sharing uses a collective pronoun (we, you, us), that person makes a definitive statement about everyone in the room, whether the member intended to or not. One of the cornerstones of our program is that everyone in the room can be where they are and believe what they believe in the moment. Using we, you, and us tells folks where they *should be* and what *they should think*.

The most important reason to speak from the "I" perspective is that the person sharing will completely own what they say. Shifting from we-you-us to I and me can profoundly affect the person sharing. The following is an example of the difference from Eric Daxon.

> I never really understood the admonition to speak from the 'I' perspective until an old-timer in a meeting said, 'You need to understand what resentment is. A resentment is...' Another old-

timer disagreed, and an argument ensued. Soon, other group members joined in. This made the meeting a very unsafe meeting.

I had a more personal lesson about this. I was in a meeting and said something that started with "we," meaning my wife and me. Specifically, I said, "We enabled our daughter." I glanced at my wife, who was shaking her head, "No." In the next meeting, I used "I." "I enabled my daughter." Two things happened. First, my wife just listened. Second, and more importantly, I took full ownership of my words. Instead of saying we enabled our daughter, I swallowed hard and said, "I enabled our daughter." Once I said it, the total weight of what I was doing fell on me like a ton of bricks. I was no longer hiding behind "we."

It is not unusual for members to slip and say we or us. If this continues or if what the family member is saying is incredibly disruptive, the coach needs to step in and kindly stop the sharing. Sometimes, just saying, "Please speak from the 'I' perspective," redirects the member. It is essential to step in if the sharing is religious or evangelistic. Another approach is to share after the person from the I perspective.

- **ENSURE GROUP MEMBERS DO NOT GIVE ADVICE OR ASK FOR ADVICE DURING THE MEETING.** Giving advice during the meeting, even by a recovery coach, makes sharing unsafe. When a family member first comes to a meeting, they have already received a lot of "advice," usually from people without experience with addiction, knowledge of recovery, or an understanding of the family's internal dynamics. This usually leads to the family member shutting down and not discussing what is happening with the "advice-givers." The same dynamic can occur in a meeting where group members are giving advice.

Giving someone unsolicited advice in a meeting is demeaning because it implies the person giving the advice has the answers and the person receiving the advice does not and cannot solve the problem on their own. There is one other harmful aspect of giving advice. Giving advice provides everyone in the room permission to not focus on themselves but to focus on someone else. This is especially the case for the person giving the advice.

- **ENSURE NO ONE ASKS QUESTIONS DURING THE MEETING.** Asking a question in a meeting is like giving advice in reverse. It carries the same pitfalls as giving advice. Group members are encouraged to ask questions or ask for advice after the meeting.

- **ENSURE THERE IS NO CROSSTALK DURING THE MEETING.** Crosstalk is talking while someone else is sharing. We ask participants to mute their microphones for virtual support group meetings until they wish to speak. An anonymous group member relayed the following example of how hurtful even harmless crosstalk can be.

> I was new to the group. I was sharing something that did not seem to be but was both personal and embarrassing. Then, someone in the group giggled. I believed they were laughing at what I said. The laughter hurt me, and I shut down immediately. The group noticed, and the giggler noticed. Later, I discovered that the person beside the giggler told a humorous, unrelated joke. The comment from the giggler was, "I did not think what you said was so personal."

In a meeting, recovery coaches must be conscious of and adhere to these rules. Our purpose in a family group 12-Step meeting is to keep the meeting safe and share from the "I" perspective. This is the one place where we can show that we do not have all the answers. This is one place where we can instill in our members that their recovery is their recovery, and they can do it without relying on a coach.

"COFFEE AFTER THE MEETING"

"Coffee," or as people in recovery sometimes call it, "The meeting after the meeting," is an integral part of the meeting. "Coffee" usually occurs at an inexpensive restaurant or in the same room as the meeting. Coffee is where members fellowship and build the bonds and trust that enhance the meeting experience. This is where family members can ask questions, get advice, or give advice. It is a place where members enjoy each other's company, laugh, and get to know each other on another level.

Coffee after the meeting offers another opportunity to learn to let go of the fear that is isolating many family members. Walking into a meeting room for the first time requires letting go of fear. Going to coffee also requires letting go of fear. It also allows family members to experience what it is like to stick with winners. Sticking with winners is not just about growing but also about having fun and building solid, trustworthy, rewarding relationships.

Recovery coaches/counselors are always at coffee. The first reason is to continue building the relationships with our members needed to make the integrated APG approach work. The second is to identify people who may need help after a meeting. Sometimes, meetings are very emotional and can leave members emotionally distraught.

Newcomer's Meeting

The primary purpose of a Newcomer's Meeting is to let the newcomers know they are not alone; there is help for them and hope for them. In addition, a Newcomer's Meeting introduces the program, meeting mechanics, and an opportunity to share their story. Newcomers are provided with meeting schedules, information about the program, and rules to keep a meeting safe, and they are asked to fill out a registration form. This is quite different from newcomer meetings in other 12-Step programs.

Volunteer group members usually run the Newcomers Meeting. There are multiple reasons why it is better not to have a recovery coach run newcomer meetings. Having a steering committee member conduct the newcomer meeting:

- PROVIDES IMMEDIATE AND INTIMATE CONTACT WITH A GROUP MEMBER WHO IS IN RECOVERY. This gives the newcomer a friendly face in the meeting, a person who could be a sponsor, and someone they can call.
- REDUCES COUNSELOR DEPENDENCE. Knowing someone in the group lets the newcomer know that others in the group, besides the counselors, can help.
- Reduces staffing requirements at a meeting.

Newcomer's 2.0

Newcomer's 2.0 is a meeting that is specific to the organizations the author's were associated with. Newcomer's 2.0 is a meeting for family group members who have been in the program for at least 30 days and have attended at least four meetings. A volunteer group member leads this meeting. The purpose of the meeting is to revisit the program's tools and allow participants to assess where they are in their program. The meeting also encourages them to continue. It also allows participants to ask questions and get more clarity on how the program works.

Speaker's Meeting

This is just like a speaker's AA meeting or any other recovery traditions. The only qualification is that the speaker must be in recovery. A speaker's meeting can be open to the public, anyone in recovery, all groups, or just one group. The speaker decides the audience. We ask the speaker to share their recovery story, focusing on their recovery. "Johnny-logs"[16] are generally less helpful than a speaker sharing their recovery story regarding their experience, love, and understanding.

Heart Meeting

The Heart Meeting is a PDAP-specific meeting where a member of the Youth Group (ages 13-17) who is in recovery shares their recovery story with the family group. It is called a Heart Meeting because, in many ways, the young person shares their heart with the family group. The purpose of this meeting is to allow parents to hear a story of hope and recovery from a member of the younger group and then to ask the speaker questions related to recovery. A group member or recovery coach facilitates the meeting and keeps the meeting safe for the speaker. Unlike a speaker's meeting, a Heart Meeting is open only

---

16 A "Johnny-log" is the family group equivalent of a "drunk-a-log." The family member just talks about what their loved one did and what the family member did in response.

to family members of the family group. This helps to ensure the safety of the speaker and family members. It also fosters openness. Here are the guidelines for the meeting:

- **THE SPEAKER IS LIMITED TO A PERSON IN THE ORGANIZATION'S YOUNGER GROUP WHO IS IN RECOVERY.** This is done for three reasons. First, it gives family members hope that their loved one can improve. Second, family members will get a feel for what their loved one is learning in the user groups. Third, just as importantly, the speaker will gain the same knowledge about the family group.

- **THE MEETING IS LIMITED TO FAMILY MEMBERS WHO HAVE ATTENDED AT LEAST FOUR MEETINGS.** The first reason is the speaker's safety. Newcomers are often raw, angry, and prone to lash out. Second, after four meetings, most of the family members in the Heart Meeting will know each other and the group's senior members. This familiarity fosters both openness and safety.

Education Meeting

As the title implies, the purpose of an education meeting is to provide information on a topic relevant to recovery from SUD or codependency. The format can range from didactic to experiential to a combination. The recovery coach chooses the topic based on the group's needs. A recovery coach usually does the education meeting. The reason for this is to ensure that the material presented is in line with the organization's approach to recovery. On those rare occasions when there is an outside speaker, the recovery coach sponsoring the event must ensure the presentation aligns with the organization's approach to recovery.

Workshops/Retreats

Workshops and retreats allow a more in-depth study of one topic. Workshops usually last up to a day. Retreats are one or more days, often over a weekend, and can address several related topics. While education is always a part of a retreat, its primary purpose is to foster connections with the coaches/counselors, other family members, and, more importantly, their Higher Power. These retreats usually include "playtime," where members can do what they like. This is another opportunity to learn how to have sober fun.

Victory Meeting

A Victory Meeting is a PDAP-specific meeting. The purpose of a Victory Meeting is to celebrate the recovery of members from all groups. Recovery staff-run Victory Meetings. These meetings recognize and celebrate key milestones in family recovery—being in the group for a year, getting a sponsor, etc. Often, these meetings include staff-run skits or other types of recovery-related entertainment. The format for a Victory Meeting varies, but the one constant is that the Victory Meeting is fun!

Parting Thoughts on Family Group Meetings

If you are working in an organization that does not provide support group meetings, this section is of limited use. We want to emphasize that none of the meetings in this section are process groups. If you are running a process group, the information here is of limited use. This applies especially to the section on keeping a meeting safe. A process group has a different purpose than a 12-Step meeting or any of the meetings discussed in this section.

CHAPTER 7

Peer Coaching/Counseling Appointments

Peer coaching/counseling appointments complement group meetings by addressing family members' individual needs. Support group meetings provide generalized recovery support for the family member and may or may not address a family member's specific needs. In addition, a family member cannot accomplish some recovery tasks in meetings. Tasks like developing a recovery plan, developing boundaries, or developing a plan to respond to a crisis are family member-specific and inappropriate for a group setting. The objectives of this chapter are to provide:

- An approach to coaching/counseling appointments consistent with the principles of recovery and tailored to meet family member needs.
- Guidance on what a peer coach should do before the first appointment.
- A process for the first appointment with a family member.

It is important to remember that a family member showing up for their first appointment is often an act of exceptional desperation and humility that will often be expressed as anger. Remember, the family member you are seeing has chosen to get into recovery. Their recovery journey is often as agonizing as the loved one's recovery journey.

General Approach

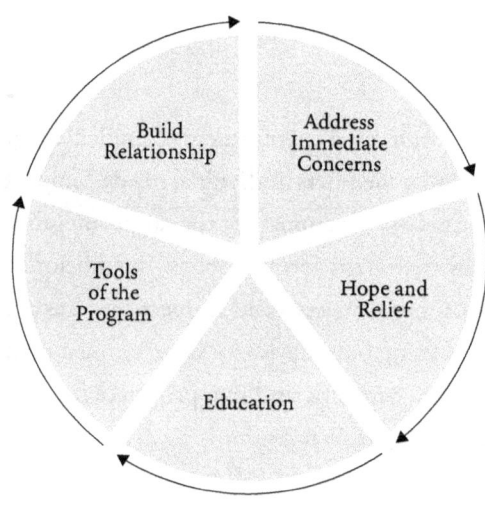

FIGURE 10. GENERAL APPROACH TO APPOINTMENTS

The general approach to appointments is shown in *Figure 10* above. Addressing immediate concerns, providing hope, and providing relief provide the emotional institutional support often needed in the initial stages of recovery. Immediate family member concerns often include how to respond to violence, mental breakdowns, threats of suicide, illegal activity, abuse of the family, and running away. It is important to address immediate needs in all appointments, but especially in the first one.

Providing hope and relief starts with the first appointment, where the coach meets the family members where they are and lets them know that they are not alone. Be alert for things the family member is doing right or for things the coach can reframe into a positive. In most cases, family members focus so much on what is going wrong that they do not see the good things they are doing.

Usually, a family member is in the preparation stage when they make an appointment. This is not always the case. Often, one member comes only to please another family member and may be in the contemplation or precontemplation stage. Education is an ongoing process, but it is essential if the family member is in the pre-contemplative or contemplative stages of recovery. Topics include the disease of SUD, codependency, enabling, family roles, recovery tools, and the impact of family involvement. Also included in education are any topics specific to a family member.

Teaching the tools of the program and holding them accountable are parts of the preparation, action, and maintenance stages of recovery. This book provides information and worksheets the recovery coach can use to teach these tools. Recovery coaches should base their decision on what tools to use and when to use them on the family member's needs.

Relationship building is a part of every appointment. This starts with ensuring the client has reasonable expectations of our role and what will occur during the appointments. Being honest, open, and willing fosters the trust needed for the relationship to benefit the family member. Judiciously sharing personal experiences is a part of relationship building but not the most important part.

Pre-Appointment

Each recovery coach has a family history that generates resentments, preconceived notions, and vulnerabilities. Hopefully, the recovery coach identified and dealt with many of these in their recovery work. However, the odds are high that some resentments, preconceived notions, and vulnerabilities will remain. If a recovery coach is aware of their issues, it is easier to recover if the family member triggers the recovery coach's resentments. If a recovery coach's personal issues hinder the family member's recovery, they need to take steps to have the family member meet with another coach.

Parents and family members can be angry, bitter, and afraid and often lash out. It is your job as a coach to learn to love—agape love—them and accept them where they are. Treating family members, especially parents, with love and compassion is easier if you can remember what the family member has been through up to this point. Typically, family members experience some or all of the following:

- **FEAR.** They know their loved one is on a path that can ruin or end their lives. Nothing they have tried seems to work. The family is also often living in fear of their loved one either because of violence, threats of violence, stealing, or their loved one's friends.

- **SHAME AND GUILT.** They blame themselves for their loved one's drug use. Society, teachers and administrators, clergy, their family, their friends, and especially loved ones often reinforce the family member's guilt and shame.

- **HELPLESSNESS.** All that they have tried has not worked. More than likely, the parents and the rest of the family are arguing over the correct course of action.

- **WORRY AND ANXIETY.** SUD impacts every aspect of the family: finances, job security, marriage, and other siblings.

- **TIRED OF ADVICE.** All their support systems have been giving them advice. In general, the advice has not helped. The advice has hurt because most advice indirectly condemns them. A good example is, "You should be harder on them." This implies that the family members were too soft in their approach.

- **BEING ALONE.** Most believe that they are alone in dealing with this issue. No one in their support system seems to be going through what they are going through. In many cases, people in their support system begin to shun them, their family, and their loved one.

- **FAMILY DISRUPTION.** SUD affects the entire family, and each family member acts out in their own way. SUD in the family can either cause marital issues or exacerbate them.

Remembering what the family member has been through, remembering what you have been through, makes it easier to accept the anger and see through the anger to what the family member is: a person deeply hurt by their loved one's SUD.

Initial Appointment

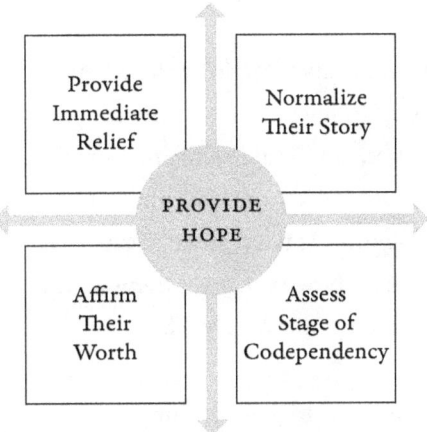

FIGURE 11. GENERAL APPROACH TO THE INITIAL APPOINTMENT

The initial appointment is crucial because it will set the stage for the remaining appointments and begin the relationship building. *Figure 11* (previous page) shows each of the objectives for the initial appointment: provide hope, normalize their story, affirm their worth, provide immediate relief, if possible, and assess the stage of codependency. The most important of these objectives is to give a sense of hope. Hope that they can get their lives back. Hope that their loved one can recover. This initial hope motivates family members to continue with a demanding, sometimes frightening process called recovery.

PROVIDE IMMEDIATE RELIEF

Education and putting in place immediate boundaries are two ways to provide immediate relief to families. Provide the basics of the disease, emphasizing how it affects the loved one's ability to make good decisions and how powerful the craving to use is. Knowing that the loved one cannot just stop helps them to view this as a disease and not a choice. Knowing the loved one is not doing this *to them* can give a great deal of relief. Provide an understanding of the 3 "C's." They did not "Cause" the disease. They cannot "Cure" the disease. They cannot "Control" the disease. This helps relieve shame, guilt, and a good deal of frustration.

It also helps to give the family something to do, especially if there is a lot of anger or grief. It is helpful to suggest they attend support group meetings, get a sponsor, attend activities, or practice self-care. Often, just telling the family member that self-care is allowed, encouraged, and helpful will bring great relief.

The boundary-setting process is a deliberate one that can take a couple of appointments to complete. However, we recommend that family members put four boundaries in place immediately. These are:

- If your loved one is high, call your coach.

- If you find drugs or paraphernalia, throw them away and call your coach.

- If there is violence or the threat of violence to family members or themselves, call 911 and leave the area.

- If your loved one is a minor and runs away, call the police and list them as a runaway.

These immediate boundaries keep the family and loved one safe during boundary-setting. Importantly, they provide relief from the most daunting challenges for a parent—not knowing what to do and fearing that what they do will harm their loved one.

NORMALIZE THEIR STORY

Normalize the family member's story by letting them know that they are not alone, their situation is not unique, and, most importantly, there is hope. Families and loved ones do recover. If appropriate, this may be a suitable time to tell them a little about your recovery story. Up to this point, most family members believe that they are alone in this, that no one else is where they are now. Knowing that they are not alone and that others have made it through this process moves them from being alone to being one of many. Hearing success stories makes them believe the process may work for them and their loved ones.

AFFIRM THEIR WORTH

In general, society, family, friends, their loved ones, and they believe that their loved one's SUD is their fault. Many have tried and failed to get their loved one to stop using substances. All are grieving the loss of their dreams for their loved ones. It is essential to accurately identify the positives for the family member and what they are doing right. If nothing else, they are sitting in an appointment seeking help.

One effective way to affirm their worth is to find positives in what they have told you in the appointment. Reframing is a sound methodology that places what they have done into recovery terminology. Here are a couple of examples:

- Reframe anger or despair as a passion for someone they dearly love.

- Point out the courage and the love it takes for them to walk through our doors and that many in their situation have not sought help.

- A parent once recounted how they told their son they would call the police, and they did call the police on their son, and that still did not work. Reframe that apparent failure into a positive by placing it into recovery terminology. "You just did one of the hardest things a parent can do. You set a boundary, and you enforced it. It takes many parents months of recovery to be able to do that. Good job!"

- During the first appointment, asking them to try the program for 90 days is important. Asking for a 90-day commitment indirectly lets them know that this is a long-term process and that family healing is not "one-and-done." It also lets them know we are in it with them for the long haul.

ASSESS STAGE OF CODEPENDENCY

Chapter 2, Substance Use Disorder, Codependency, and Family Roles, discusses the characteristics of each of the four stages of codependency. The assessment aims to determine if the family member needs help from allied professionals such as psychiatrists, psychologists, or therapists. It is not unusual for family members in Stage 3 or Stage 4 Codependency to suffer from anxiety, depression, or other stress-related illnesses. These illnesses may require specialized treatment from mental health professionals.

Follow-up Appointments

There is no set pattern for follow-up appointments. Since most adult family members have little idea of what they need, a good approach is to identify two or three areas and ask the family members which they want to address first. It would seem natural to go right into the recovery planning, but experience has shown that most families need some stability and knowledge before the recovery planning process is effective. As always, if a family member desires to move right into recovery planning, we move into recovery planning. Chapter 8, Family Member Recovery Plan, provides guidance for developing a family member's recovery plan.

Parting Thoughts on Appointments with Family Members

It is essential to meet the family members where they are in the moment. Simply asking how the family member is doing is the best way to find out where the family member is. Sometimes, the family member is in a good place, and the appointment can proceed as planned. Sometimes, the family member is so distraught that they need to dump. If this is the case, let them dump, and then help them understand the issues plaguing them and assist their transition to talking about recovery. Asking open-ended questions directed at a discrepancy in the discussion or non-recovery beliefs is an effective method to guide the family member toward viewing the events through a recovery lens.

In one case, a client bitterly complained about his wife enforcing a boundary their adult child had crossed. The consequence of crossing the boundary was that the adult child needed to move out of the house. The client's anger at his wife was visceral. The coach listened and then asked him to delineate the disagreement precisely. The client started by saying, "She does not want to enforce the boundary!" The coach knew this was not the case and asked, "Your wife does not want your child to leave? Didn't you say earlier that she agreed the child needed to leave?" The client responded sheepishly, "Well, yes, but my wife does not want to help our child move her stuff out, and I do." The coach replied, "So you both agree on the important thing, but you are arguing over how she will move out? Does that seem reasonable? Can you control what your wife does? Can she control what you do?" The relief and the guilt on the client's face were apparent. He realized he and his wife agreed on the important thing: the adult child must leave home. He realized he could not control his wife, and she could not control him. He could do it his way, and she could do it hers.

The story above is Eric's. The other thing that made Eric's peer coach so effective was her genuine empathy. In Eric's words:

> I knew she understood what I was saying because she summarized things often during our appointments. She gave me the affirmations I needed—I was enforcing a hard boundary, I was using my recovery tools (getting an appointment), and I loved my child. Her last two questions reinforced the recovery principle that I could only control my actions. The discussion led me to understand that my two most prominent character defects—pride and fear—were behind my anger. The pride: "I was right." The fear: "If you do not do it my way, my child will die." Finally, the counselor reminded me that I do not control outcomes; our Higher Power does.

Eric's peer coach displayed empathy, used active listening, and confronted Eric with love and empathy. Here are a couple of other suggestions for how to talk to family members:

- **DO NOT "SHOULD" ALL OVER THEM.** Refrain from telling a family member what they should do. When a family member comes in for help, well-meaning family and friends have already been "shoulding" all over them.

- **NEW TOOLS.** Frame recovery as a process of acquiring the parenting tools needed to deal with a loved one with SUD. In most cases, the parent/guardian's approach worked for other siblings and the loved one until SUD entered the picture. Telling a parent/guardian they could not use a tool they did not have is a way to reduce unwarranted guilt.

- **FALL IN AGAPE LOVE WITH THE FAMILY MEMBER.** This is important. One of our core values is unconditional love and emoting that agape love to the family member. Spend some time before the appointment in prayer for the family member. Pray that your Higher Power gives them all the good things in life.

CHAPTER 8

Family Member Recovery Plan

Like their loved ones, family members need a recovery plan. Like their loved one's recovery plan, theirs is based on mind, body, and spirit. Also, like their loved one, their plan is holistic and person-driven. The family member is the planner and the decision-maker in this process. The recovery coach's role is to provide the planning tools, be an honest broker, serve as the client's advocate, and identify and help obtain the resources the family members need. The purpose of this chapter is to assist in that planning process by:

- Providing an understanding of some impediments preventing a family member from engaging in recovery planning.

- Providing a recovery planning approach that covers all the domains of recovery.

- Providing approaches to overcome the impediments to planning.

There are more detailed recovery planning approaches. The Wellness Recovery Action Plan is an example process that covers all four SAMHSA domains in detail (Copland 2018).

Recovery Plan Development

Figure 12 below shows our approach to developing a family member's recovery plan. The approach is standard except for the first component—restoring hope. There are times when a family member's guilt, depression, or hopelessness are so pervasive that it is difficult for them to contemplate recovery, let alone develop a recovery plan. The purpose of Appendix A: Recovery Plan Preparation, is, in part, to help a family member regain the hope needed to move forward. The approach in the appendix seeks to remind the family members of their strengths and their passions and that life once was and can be joy-filled again.

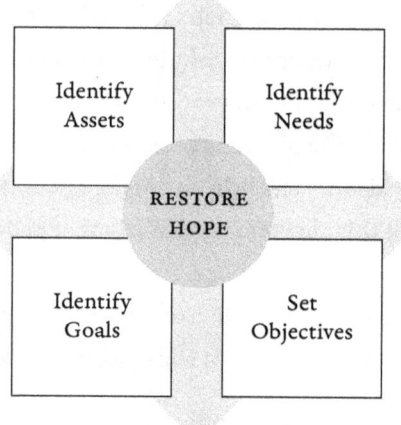

FIGURE 12. PROCESS FOR DEVELOPING A RECOVERY PLAN

Identifying assets, needs, and goals and setting objectives are standard steps to most plan development processes. Appendix B: Codependency Recovery Plan is a tool to assist the family member in completing each of these steps. Two more appendices deal with recovery plan development. The first is Appendix C: Plan for Enjoyment and Fun. Enjoyment and fun are so crucial to the integrated APG approach that we ask family members to develop plans to have fun with their friends, families, spouse/significant others, and alone. All of these relationships are important for recovery, and fun strengthens the bonds in each of them.

The second is Appendix D: Codependency Relapse Prevention and Relapse Recovery Plan. Like the loved one, codependents relapse. Planning to prevent a relapse and having a plan to recover from a relapse reduces the risk of relapse and hastens recovery from a relapse. Each of these appendices is discussed in detail in the following sections.

Using Appendix A: Recovery Plan Preparation

Helping a family member get ready for recovery planning starts with bringing hope by first reminding them of their strengths, gifts, talents, accomplishments, and support systems. Reminding family members of their strengths is important because it is common for parents and family members to forget how capable they are and come to believe they are helpless. Second, it reminds them of the joy, happiness, and satisfaction they have already had. It is common for family members to forget the good times, the satisfying times in their lives. Forgetting the good times often gives the family member a feeling of helpless hopelessness that can impede or thwart recovery planning.

REMEMBERING THE GOOD TIMES

The first series of questions in Appendix A, Recovery Plan Preparation, reminds the family member of the good times. QUESTIONS 1 and 2 ask the family member to describe four good memories from their past in sufficient detail so that someone else could live them. This is getting them to remember that life was once good. Sometimes, the client will say that they cannot remember or never had good times. Gently probe or bring up things the family member said in appointments or meetings. Asking about significant life events like getting married or the birth of a child can bring up memories of these events or spark memories of other joyous events. Also, ask about seemingly minor events. Examples of seemingly insignificant events in the appendix include an unexpected day off from school or eating a favorite food. Sometimes, the family members cannot remember good times in their lives. This is especially true for family members in Stage 4 Codependency. These family members may need more help than a recovery coach can provide and may need to be referred to an allied health professional.

QUESTION 3 concerns remembering and describing when the family member felt calm and anxiety-free. Like remembering the good times, family members can have trouble remembering when they felt relaxed and anxiety-free. Like the good times, calm events can be relatively simple events. Joanne Daxon tells the following story, which is an excellent example of this question. "I remember going to church with my grandfather when I was a young girl. I enjoyed the quiet in church and felt close to my grandfather. On the way home, we stopped at a bakery, and the baker always gave me a sugar cookie. The sugar cookie made me feel special."

QUESTION 4 asks the family member to try to review the moments of calm and then write down the good, positive thoughts that come to mind. If the family member has difficulty with this, ask them to try remembering the smells and the sounds associated with the event. For Joanne, it was the smell of the bakery and the sound of her grandfather's voice. Ask about anything they might have felt. Was the wind blowing? Was it cold or hot? Did someone's hand feel rough or smooth as they held their hand?

QUESTION 5 asks the family member to recognize and describe critical accomplishments. The key is not the enormity of the task but that the family member was proud of what he/she did. These can be simple things like learning to bait a hook, riding a bike, finally jumping off the high dive, or someone the family member respects saying, "Good job." They can be not-so-simple things: graduating, getting an award or promotion, figuring out a challenging problem, or completing an arduous task.

QUESTION 6 moves from remembering the past to thinking about the present by asking the family members what interests them and what they enjoy doing. The QUESTION 6 table lists several activities to jog the family member's memory and spaces to add what may be missing. This is the preparatory work for doing the enjoyment and fun plan in Appendix C. This question is designed to start the family members thinking about what they enjoy doing. Enjoyment is something most family members have not thought about since SUD entered their lives. It also gives the recovery coach an understanding of the activities that bring joy to the family member.

Similarly, QUESTION 7 asks them to circle or write about the tasks or activities they are good at. This task has two extremes—circling none or circling a great many. If the family member struggles to find anything to select, use the information gained in appointments and meetings to suggest activities they enjoy and areas where their strengths may lie. If the family member circles a large number, ask the family member to choose the top five.

QUESTION 8 is about identifying other organizations with which the family member is involved. The primary purpose of this question is to remind the family members that other organizations can support them.

QUESTION 9 asks the family member to identify the good things they have in their lives. The intent here is to help them remember and focus on what is going right in their lives. This also helps to identify areas in their lives that they may need to work on.

QUESTION 10 asks the family member to identify people who will foster the family member's recovery. In colloquial terms, we call these people "winners." This process has two outcomes. First, it identifies the people who will aid the family member in their recovery. Second and equally importantly, it identifies the people that will hamper the family member's recovery. The family member needs to understand three concepts about winners.

- A WINNER FOR THE FAMILY MEMBER IS SOMEONE WHO ENCOURAGES OR FACILITATES THEIR RECOVERY. Being or not being a winner is about whether a person's faults or strengths encourage or discourage the family member's recovery. Someone who is not a winner for the family member does not mean that they are a terrible person. It just means the person's faults or strengths hinder the family member's recovery.

- BEING A WINNER CAN BE SITUATIONALLY DEPENDENT. A family member can be a winner for you in every aspect except discussions about your loved one's recovery. Someone can be a winner for you, except when they are drinking.

- SOME ARE NOT WINNERS IN ALL SITUATIONS. In some cases, the person's personality is so antithetical to the family member's recovery that they cannot be around them at all. Again, this does not mean he is a bad person. It just means his weaknesses and strengths hinder the family member's recovery.

An anonymous family group member described a winner in this way:

I heard my first explanation of a 'winner' in 1997 at a family group meeting. The counselor talked about a friend who was a winner in every aspect of his recovery except one—shopping in a sporting goods store. Both loved the outdoors; both loved shopping at sporting goods stores; both had a spending addiction. If they shopped at a sporting goods store together, they would egg each other on and end up metaphorically "buying the store out." This man was a winner in every other aspect of the counselor's life—drug use, relationships, working a program. They could not shop at a sporting goods store together.

Eric has his own "winner" story. As Eric states:

> I had a sponsee that I liked. We had a lot in common: similar personalities, similar family situations, similar likes, similar dislikes, and similar marriages. We used to meet at a restaurant, eat, do step-work, and .... begin complaining about our wives. The conversation inevitably turned to gossiping about our wives whenever we were together. I liked him, and we were winners for each other except when we talked about our wives.

Using Appendix B: Codependency Recovery Plan

Appendix B provides a framework for family members to develop their recovery plan. QUESTION 1 in Appendix B is essential, "Is there anything you need to work on right now?" Many times, some issues need to be immediately addressed. If this is the case, suspend the recovery plan development process and work to help solve the pressing problem. If the family member just lost their job and wants help getting a new job, the task becomes assisting them.

If a loved one has reached the point where they need inpatient treatment, the task becomes helping them get the loved one into treatment.

NEEDS ASSESSMENT

The appendix uses *Table 1, Needs Assessment,* on page 294, to determine the gaps preventing a family member from living their best life. The table has a series of positive statements about mind, body, spirit, and recovery. QUESTION 2 starts the needs assessment by asking the family member to rate their agreement with the statements in the table on a 1 to 7 scale. Where 1 is strongly disagree, 2 is disagree, 3 is slightly disagree, 4 is neither agree nor disagree, 5 is slightly agree, 6 is agree, and 7 is strongly agree. The lower the score, the more the family member needs to work on the area of their life indicated by the statement. Ask the family member to rate all the statements first and then go back and determine which ones they want to work on now.

GOAL DEVELOPMENT

QUESTION 3 starts the goal-setting process by asking the family member to review the needs assessment and select up to three that they want to work on now. The question asks the family member to focus on statements they disagreed with—those rated 1, 2, 3, or 4. Further, if they want to work on areas they agreed with—rated 5, 6, or 7- they must discuss those with their recovery coach. A family member may want to work on a statement they agree with for several reasons. First, this is an essential area in their lives, and they want to improve it further. Second, the family member is in denial, and they are starting to see reality. Third, and most likely, there is another unresolved issue related to the statement. For example, a family group member strongly agreed with a statement about their faith community but still wanted to work on it because there were parts of his faith life that he wanted to explore more deeply. As he delved into the development of his action plan, he realized that he had a deep resentment against his church because, years ago, the church shunned his loved one. The real issue for this father was resentment.

Other times, a family member's answers can indicate a gap in one area, but it is actually in another area of their lives. In one case, a family member's needs inventory showed a severe gap in their relationship with their Higher Power. The recovery coach probed and found that the family member had a good relationship with his Higher Power but was holding on to a debilitating resentment against a sibling. The family member did not need to work on his relationship with his Higher Power but needed to work on forgiveness.

QUESTION 4 asks the family member to develop separate action plans to fill the gaps they want to work on now using *Table 2, Action Plan Template,* on page 298. The first step is for the family member to delineate the action plan's goal. How do they want their current life to change? The goal needs to be specific, realistic, and something they can do. Sometimes, the statements in the needs assessment are straightforward and identify a definitive finite gap. For example, "I have a sponsor and am working with a sponsor." Disagreement indicates that the family member does not have a sponsor or has one and is not working with them. The goal becomes either finding a sponsor or starting to work with their sponsor.

Some statements are more general and do not indicate a specific gap. For example, a family member strongly disagrees with the statement, "I feel safe in my home." The gap is a feeling of being unsafe, but the family member needs to articulate what is making the home dangerous before they can develop an actionable goal or goals. If the home is unsafe because of severe structural issues, the goal becomes fixing it or moving out. If it is the violent behavior of a family member, the goal becomes putting boundaries in place to protect the family member and the rest of the family.

ROADBLOCKS AND STRENGTHS

Roadblocks are what the name implies. They are hindering the family member's ability to accomplish their goal. Roadblocks can be gaps in the family member's resources. These could include not having transportation, childcare, shelter, medical/dental insurance, food, or clothing. They can also be intangible, like fear, uncontrolled anger, resentment, denial, no Higher Power, non-recovery beliefs, guilt/shame, or debilitating grief. Filling tangible resource gaps is straightforward because the goal and the action steps are usually well-defined. Filling the intangible gaps is not as well defined because the endpoints are often subjective. Chapter 9, Barriers to Recovery, provides tools for the recovery coach to overcome these intangible barriers.

Strengths are those family member attributes or resources that will contribute to overcoming the roadblocks and attaining the goal. The family member's work in the recovery plan preparation should help the family member and the recovery coach identify their strengths. Identifying strengths brings hope to the family members and guides the plan's development to attain the goal.

OBJECTIVES

Objectives are specific tasks the family member needs to complete to attain their goal. Objectives should be small, concrete, measurable, attainable, and time-limited actions to attain the goal. The final part of developing objectives is identifying who will hold the family member accountable. Often, this is a sponsor, recovery coach, or a friend. The person holding accountability can be another family member, but we do not recommend this. It is better to have an objective third party responsible for accountability. Naming a specific person(s) for accountability allows the recovery coach to ensure that the named-person is a winner for the family member in that area. Asking an overly critical person for accountability is likely more hurtful than helpful for goal accomplishment.

Using Appendix C: Plan for Enjoyment and Fun

Enjoyment and fun are essential to family member recovery because enjoyment and fun are often the first casualties when SUD strikes a family. The approach uses fun to help repair three of the most significant relationships the family member has: their relationship with themselves, their relationship with their significant other, and their relationship with their family and friends. Appendix C: Plan for Enjoyment and Fun has three sections corresponding to the three essential relationships.

Each of the three sections in the appendix takes the client through the same processes—remembering past fun, selecting activities, evaluating the activity, and then selecting three things they would like to do soon.

QUESTION 1 in each of the three sections of the worksheet reminds the family member that there were times when they had fun alone, with their significant other, and with family and friends. More importantly, it is to remind them what it feels like to have fun.

QUESTION 2 in the three sections asks the client to circle the things they enjoy doing alone, with their significant other, or with friends. There are spaces in each of the tables to add activities that are not listed.

QUESTIONS 3 and 4 in each of the three sections ask the client to reexamine the circled items and identify those activities that leave them refreshed and revived. As noted in QUESTION 3, some activities leave one feeling worse. Social media is a good example, and computer games are another example.

The following section is the actual enjoyment and fun plan. Critical points for a recovery coach here are:

- Make sure the activities are restorative for the family member.
- Ensure the plan is attainable and reasonable.
- Help the client set reasonable dates for doing the task.

Using Appendix D: Codependency Relapse Prevention and Relapse Recovery Plan

Like a substance user's relapse, a codependent relapse starts well before the relapse occurs. Building Up to Drinking and Drugging or BUDD'ing is the term used for the period before relapse for substance users. Like substance users, codependents also BUDD before a relapse. While a substance user may not be aware they are BUDD'ing, they know when they have relapsed because they are using substances again. However, unlike substance users, codependents often do not see that they are relapsing because there is often no clear indicator of relapse.

The worksheet in this appendix helps a family member do two things. The first is to recognize when they are BUDD'ing and when they are relapsing. The second is to develop a plan to prevent or recover from a relapse in progress. The worksheet has three sections, and the following is a discussion of each.

FEELINGS, BEHAVIORAL CHANGES, AND TRIGGERS THAT WARN OF IMPENDING RELAPSE

The approach to identifying the family member's BUDD'ing warning signs is reexamining those times when the family member had an overwhelming desire to withdraw or an irresistible urge to rescue, punish, enable, or control the loved one. If the family member is in recovery, this is a relapse. If not, this is just a bad day. QUESTION 1 on page 310 starts the process by asking the family member to identify a past relapse (or terrible day) and describe what happened in detail. The purpose of this question is to bring the event into focus for the family member and to give the recovery coach a clear understanding of what happened.

QUESTION 2 asks about the family member's feelings, physical health, and mental health before the relapse. Surprisingly, good feelings, such as hope, can be a prelude to a relapse. Unrealistic hope, like believing the loved one will never use substances again after treatment, can rapidly turn into rage and deep resentment if the loved one relapses.

QUESTIONS 3 and 4 specifically address the family member's recovery program. Roy, a younger group recovery coach, always asked relapsing teens, "What part of your program did you stop doing?" Invariably, the teen stopped one or more aspects of their program before the relapse. The same can be true for family members. QUESTION 4 deals specifically with the family member's relationship with their Higher Power. Higher Power is a separate question because of the importance of this relationship in preventing relapse and how often family members discount the importance of this relationship in avoiding relapse.

QUESTION 5 asks the family member to think about the state of their significant relationships before the relapse. Turmoil with a spouse/significant other can erode a family member's resilience, increasing their vulnerability to a codependent relapse. The recovery coach should not discount the impact of turmoil with a boss, pastor, sponsor, or another spiritual advisor on the codependent sobriety of a family member. QUESTIONS 6 and 7 ask the family member to recall significant life events and triggers before the relapse.

The final question in this section (QUESTION 8) asks the family member to remember other relapses or "terrible days" and select the common characteristics. Determining causality is not important at this point. Whether the feeling, event, ailment, or trigger caused the relapse is not as significant as the family member recognizing that these signs are a warning that the family member is BUDD'ing. They can take action to prevent the codependent relapse.

KNOWING WHEN YOU ARE RELAPSING

As already mentioned, often, a family member will not know that they are in a codependent relapse. The purpose of this section of the worksheet is to use the remembered relapses to identify the characteristics of their codependent relapse. The questions in this section address the following: How did the family member react when things went wrong? What did the family member feel during the relapse? What did other people say about the family member during the relapse? How did other people react to the family member during the family member's relapse? The purpose of this is to give the family members signposts to alert them that they are in relapse and need to activate their relapse recovery plan.

STOPPING A CODEPENDENT RELAPSE BEFORE OR DURING THE RELAPSE

The plan to prevent or stop a codependent relapse has two parts. The first part is asking the family member the steps that they are going to take when the family member realizes they are either BUDD'ing or are in relapse. The second and more important part is asking the family member to write down the steps they want others to take to stop the family member's BUDD'ing or relapse. Then, specify who they want to take these steps and then notify these people. Giving people permission to intervene makes it more likely that the person will intervene and makes it much more likely that the family member will listen to the intervention.

Parting Thoughts on Family Member Recovery Planning

The most important concept for a peer recovery coach is remembering that it is the family member's recovery plan. It is family member-driven and family member-approved. Second, it is important to ask at the beginning of each appointment if there is an issue the family member wants to address immediately. If you are working on the enjoyment plan and the family member wants to address boundaries—work on boundaries.

When coaching the family member in the development of their recovery plan, there are several essential things to keep in mind:

- RESTORE HOPE FIRST. The first step in the family recovery planning process is instilling a sense of hope, a feeling that they deserve recovery, and a belief that family recovery does work. Once hope is restored, the family member can develop an effective recovery plan.

- THE POWER OF SETTING PRIORITIES: IT'S THE FAMILY MEMBER'S PREROGATIVE. Recovery is not about the coach's agenda but about the client's needs and goals. As recovery coaches, we identify inconsistencies, educate, and offer options, but the family member ultimately sets the course.

- ADDRESS THE PROBLEMS THAT ARE IMPORTANT TO THE CLIENT. The client might be in Stage 4 Codependency and needs professional help but wants help getting a job and nothing else. The task is developing a plan for the client to get a job. Part of the plan for getting a job may be addressing the family member's mental health needs.

- **GIVE ADVICE SPARINGLY.** Family members in Stage 1 and 2 codependency are less likely to ask for advice than family members in Stage 3 or 4 codependency. In our experience, family members usually know what they need to do but are unwilling to do it. Working through options for the next steps is an effective way for them to clear away what is blocking their ability to see their next steps. There are exceptions. The client is in Stage 4. Codependency is an exception. In this stage, rational thought is often difficult, and the family member frequently needs professional assistance.

- **PROGRESS IN RECOVERY LEADS TO CHANGES IN THE PLAN.** It is not unusual for a family member to not buy into the complete program. This is especially true when getting a sponsor. As the client works on their program, the need for each part of the program becomes clearer. Sponsorship—getting and being a sponsor—is a good example. Many are hesitant to do it because they do not see the value. This changes as they hear others talk about the impact getting a sponsor and sponsoring others had on their lives.

- **CONFRONT THE CLIENT WHEN NECESSARY.** Peer coaches are truth-tellers.

- **IDENTIFY THE NEED FOR ADDITIONAL SUPPORT AND ASSIST IN GAINING THE NEEDED HELP.** Clients in Stage 3 or, especially, Stage 4 codependency often need professional help to deal with mental illness, past trauma, currently occurring trauma, relationship issues, and family issues. Relay your concerns to the client and help them to attain the needed assistance. Seek the aid of your supervisor immediately if you become aware of suicidal ideation, child abuse, or elder abuse.

There are exceptions to each of the following characteristics, but generally, these apply mainly to parents or guardians entering recovery.

- **FAMILY MEMBERS ARE GUILT AND SHAME-STRICKEN.** Family members feel guilt and sometimes shame because they are "that family." The family has a drug addict. Friends, coworkers, and pastors will try to "help them understand where the family went wrong." Sometimes, support groups will ostracize the family. In one case, a church group member emailed the other members of the group, blaming a teen's drug use on the parents' divorce. Then, the church barred the teen from church activities. Thankfully, stories like this are becoming increasingly rare but still occur.

- **FAMILY MEMBERS ARE ANGRY AND OFTEN ARGUE.** Family members, especially parents/guardians, are desperate to save their loved ones from SUD, but nothing they do works. The parent/guardians ground the loved one so the loved one uses substances in their room or the loved one sneaks out. The family member yells, hoping to get through to the loved one, and the loved one yells back. They take the phone, and the loved one steals it or borrows a phone from a friend. After each failed attempt to stop drug use, anger, shame, and mortal fear grow until they consume the family member, the family, and the loved one. Eric and Joanne have a story in which they disagreed on handling their loved one. Eric wanted to say yes, and Joanne wanted to say no. They got angry with each other, and they argued over who was right. The following week, the same situation arose. Eric wanted to say no this time, and Joanne wanted to say yes. They got angry with each other, and they argued.

Early in recovery, the only constants with Eric and Joanne were anger and arguments over what to do.

- **FAMILY MEMBERS FORGET THAT THERE WERE EVER GOOD TIMES.** Living in this morass makes it difficult for a family member to believe he can get his life back. Depending on the family member's stage in codependency, the family member may come to think that they deserve the misery they are in. This is true in Stage 3—Self-will is working; normal relationship tools are failing - and especially true in Stage 4—Self-will is failing; normal relationship tools are failing.

PART III

Recovery Tools

Part III of the tool chest addresses the roadblocks that hinder a family member's recovery and provides specific tools to aid a peer recovery coach working with family members. Chapter 9, Barriers to Recovery, discusses the significant hindrances to family member recovery and provides the peer recovery coach with suggestions for using recovery tools to overcome these barriers. Chapter 10 through Chapter 16 have detailed discussions of common recovery tools.

CHAPTER 10, Boundaries for Families Dealing with Substance Use Disorder, provides an approach to assist family members in setting boundaries with their loved ones and others if required. It has example boundaries that a recovery coach can use to give family members an idea of a good boundary. The ROAD tool discussed in CHAPTER 11, Resent, Own, Appreciate, Demand (ROAD) Tool, is a companion tool for boundaries. The ROAD tool provides a process that helps transform a boundary from being a punishment to being a way to support the family and the loved one.

CHAPTER 12 discusses the Living in the Moment tool. The ability to "live in the moment" provides a method for the family to enjoy peaceful moments by teaching the family members to live in the present and not the past and especially not the future.

CHAPTER 13, Strengthening a Relationship with God, has four tools intended to assist a family member in improving their conscious contact with their Higher Power. These include gratitude lists, a worksheet that focuses on the prayers in the AA Big Book, a worksheet to improve a family member's prayer and meditation, and writing a letter to God and then writing God's response to the letter.

CHAPTER 14, Moving from Non-recovery Beliefs to Recovery Beliefs, has a tool that allows a family member to delve into their beliefs about recovery and identify recovery and non-recovery beliefs. The chapter provides a process to encourage the adoption of recovery beliefs. The final two chapters offer tools to deal with guilt/shame (CHAPTER 15) and tools to help the grieving process (CHAPTER 16).

Like CHAPTER 8, CHAPTER 10 through CHAPTER 16 have one or more worksheets the peer recovery coach can give the family member. When a chapter has a worksheet, the chapter provides instructions on how to use the worksheet. APPENDIX E: Suggested Reading List, has a list of books for family members and peer recovery coaches.

CHAPTER 9

Barriers to Recovery

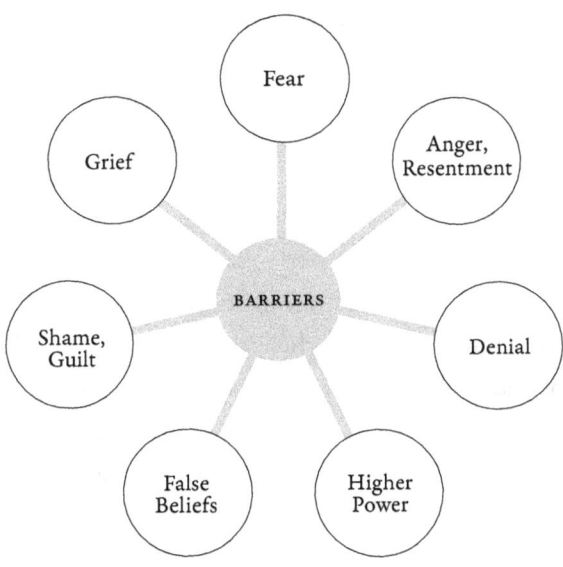

FIGURE 13. BARRIERS TO FAMILY MEMBER RECOVERY

Multiple barriers can hinder a family member's ability to recover from codependency. Some of these are due to the nature of SUD, some are due to the nature of codependency, and some are due to the loved one, but the most significant barriers are related to the family member. This chapter aims to discuss the significant hindrances to a family member's recovery and suggest tools to help the family member overcome these roadblocks. *Figure 13* (previous page) shows the main barriers to family member recovery: fear, anger and resentment, denial, lack of trust in a Higher Power, false beliefs, shame/guilt, and grief. Each of these can hinder or block a family member's recovery. The objectives of this chapter are to:

- Describe the barriers to family member recovery in a way that provides an intellectual and emotional understanding.

- Provide recommendations for the tools that might help the family member overcome the barriers.

Fear

It is hard to overstate the fear family members have when a loved one has SUD. First, the family member's fear is *for* their loved one. They fear that their loved one will die from an overdose, die from the violence associated with drug use or related accidental death (e.g., a car accident), or that human traffickers will force their loved one into human slavery. Family members fear their loved one will commit crimes that result in prison. Family members fear their loved one will commit suicide.

The next series of fears for their loved one may seem like *non-sequiturs*, given the seriousness of the previous fears, but they are not. Family members, especially parents/guardians, fear their loved one will not graduate high school on time. To some, not graduating on time may seem a trivial fear, but it is not. Family members fear their loved one will lose a job, lose a house, or get kicked off a sports team. The power of this fear and the accompanying desperation is not easy to comprehend unless you have been through it.

Second only to the fear for their loved one is fear *of their loved one*. Families fear the loved one's physical violence, either directed against them or the family's property. In one instance, a dad put a deadbolt on his youngest son's door because he was afraid of what the loved one might do to his youngest son. In another example, a loved one's drug dealer sprayed the family's house with bullets. A loved one's anger often leads to smashed doors, holes in walls, broken furniture, and broken heirlooms. It is common for family members to put locks on bedroom doors to prevent their loved ones from stealing their jewelry, electronics, or clothes. Many families are living with their loved one's verbal abuse.

Living in this kind of fear can terrorize family members to the point that they are constantly walking on eggshells, worried that they might say something to set their loved one off. The family members can become hypervigilant to the point that they neglect themselves and the rest of the family. Family members will say "yes" to the loved one when the family member knows the correct answer is "no." Agreeing to something that a family member knows is wrong can lead to guilt, shame, anxiety, and eventually depression.

An additional fear is fear of criticism and blame by extended family, friends, clergy, and medical professionals. Well-meaning family and friends who are not familiar with SUD or recovery will indirectly criticize by offering advice and telling family members what they should do. This advice is often conflicting and usually enables the loved one. Well-meaning clergy and professionals will go through the laundry list of things to ensure you raise good children, implying the family member failed in one of these areas.

Overcoming these and other fears that hinder recovery can be a long-term process. Below are tools that are usually helpful in overcoming fear.

- **EDUCATION.** Educating family members on SUD, codependency, enabling, and family dynamics provides the factual foundation needed to get the "head" on board. This is where a family member understands that recovery and recovery practices are the right things to do. It provides the family member with the tools needed to blunt the fear of criticism. It is much easier to take criticism when you know it is wrong. Understanding the recovery process for both SUD and codependency normalizes what they are going through. Chapter 2 above discusses SUD and codependency. Chapter 3 discusses the recovery process.

- **APPOINTMENTS.** Appointments will help with all the roadblocks. Appointments are under fear because one antidote to fear is a relationship with a trustworthy person who has overcome the fears the family member is facing. Chapter 7, Peer Coaching/Counseling Appointments, guides the conduct of the first and follow-up appointments.

- **SUPPORT GROUP MEETINGS AND STEP-WORK.** Fear is easier to overcome when you are not going through it alone. Support group meetings and step-work provide the fellowship, encouragement, emotional support, and understanding needed to work a good recovery program.

- **FUN.** As discussed in Chapter 5 above, fun is a core aspect of this culture, and learning to have fun again, helps overcome fear.

- **BOUNDARIES.** Boundaries reduce the fear of not knowing what to do in response to the loved one's actions. Chapter 10, Boundaries for Families Dealing with Substance Use Disorder, has a detailed discussion of the boundary-setting process. Knowing what to do can bring immediate relief from the fear of not knowing what to do.

- **LIVING IN THE MOMENT.** There are many acronyms for fear. One of them is "future events appearing real." Often, a family member is in misery, not just thinking about catastrophic events that might occur but living as if these potential future events will occur. This fear of a future event that might or might not happen prevents the family member from enjoying those enjoyable moments.

Chapter 12, Living in the Moment, is a tool that helps family members live in the moment.

- **HIGHER POWER.** A strong belief in a Higher Power is the most effective antidote to fear. Chapter 13, Strengthening a Relationship with God, has methods and tools to aid a family member in improving their relationship with their Higher Power.

Anger, Resentments

Anger and resentment fuel codependency. They also provide the energy needed in Stage 1 and Stage 2 codependency to continue a course of self-will using tools that are not working. Eventually, the self-will tank will run dry, and then the anger and resentment fuel the anxiety and depression that accompany Stage 3 and Stage 4 Codependency. A family member can direct their anger at the loved one, the loved one's dealer, or the world. Some family members will blame the world, the government, or current laws for their loved one's substance use, and they go on a crusade to change things. They may also blame the lack of resources to fight substance use and try to influence federal, state, and local governments; blame the schools and try to get new school policies; blame the drug dealers and try to get them arrested. This kind of activism is often good, sometimes destructive, but does not help the family members recover from codependency.

It is important to remember that anger and resentment are often just defense mechanisms protecting a vulnerable family member from dealing with something they never imagined would happen to their family. It is also important to remember that a family member being angry with their loved one does not mean they do not love their loved one. Tools that can assist in dealing with family member anger and resentment include:

- STEP-WORK. One of the main objectives of step-work is to deal with anger and resentment. Working with a sponsor gives the family member a safe person to vent to and provides a proven methodology to deal with resentments.

- SUPPORT GROUP MEETINGS. Support group meetings let family members know they are not alone in their anger. More importantly, these meetings show how others have worked through anger and resentment and regained their lives. Support group meetings also provide a head and a heart-understanding that you can love someone and be angry at them.

- EDUCATION. Often, anger is caused by the false belief that the loved one is using substances to hurt the family member. It is common to hear a family member ask, "How could he do this to me?" The loved one's substance use usually has nothing to do with the family member.

- APPOINTMENTS. Appointments will help with all the roadblocks. Appointments provide a safe place for family members to vent their anger and resentment. An appointment also allows the recovery coach to reframe the anger and help the family member work through the resentments blocking the recovery process. The ROAD tool, discussed in Chapter 11, assists in this process.

- PROFESSIONAL HELP. Often, anger is a symptom of an underlying mental health issue that needs more help than a recovery coach can provide.

Denial

Denial is both a shield and a hindrance. It shields family members and keeps them safe from things they cannot handle. This is a good thing in early recovery. However, in later recovery, it is a hindrance because it prevents effectively dealing with the actual issues confronting them and their families. In general, family member denial starts with denying that their loved one has a substance use problem. Then, it often moves to denying that the family member needs help.

FAMILY MEMBER DENYING THE LOVED ONE NEEDS HELP

It is important to remember that denial is an effective defense mechanism for the family member who cannot cope with knowing their loved one has SUD—a life-threatening and still shame-producing disease. At a point in time, denial is doing more harm than good for the family member, the family, and the loved one. Rick and Julie's story is an excellent example of a family member in denial. Rick and Julie were family group members whose daughter had SUD. Julie understood and accepted what was happening to their daughter from the outset. On the other hand, Rick needed to stay in denial for a while. They agreed to use their story but asked us to use fictitious names.

As Rick put it, "All I wanted out of life was a good family and a good marriage. Good families do not have substance use issues." He was in denial that his daughter used drugs at all. When it became apparent that his daughter was using drugs, Rick shifted to, "It is just a phase. She does not have a problem. She will grow out of it." Rick's daughter needed inpatient care. His wife, Julie, and his daughter's counselor waited until he was on a business trip to take their daughter to a treatment facility. Julie and the counselor did this because they knew Rick would oppose this. Rick said he did not want his daughter to go to treatment because he did not want her labeled as a person with an addiction. His pride hindered his ability to see reality.

Rick knew about the disease of SUD. He knew what the signs were. His pride, both in his family and himself, kept Rick in denial until one of his daughter's treatment counselors confronted him directly. "Rick, your daughter is an addict and needs help." As he described this encounter, "I was initially angry, then sad. As the truth of what the counselor said set in, I remembered what so many people in my family group said about denial and the disease. I knew the counselor was right, and I accepted it."

Rick's moving from denial to understanding was a gradual process that started with Rick attending family group meetings. Rick heard other parents talk about their denial and what brought them out of denial. He heard other family members talk about how their loved one was acting. It was beginning to sink in, but as Rick said, "For the first four months of going to meetings, I was expecting one of the counselors to tap me on the shoulder and tell me I did not need to be there. My kid was experimenting."

There are no quick fixes for this denial. It is usually a gradual process. The tools listed below can help:

- **EDUCATION.** As described in Rick's story, having a good understanding of the disease of addiction and the concurrent signs and symptoms is the starting point for overcoming denial. Using the relationship model of addiction discussed in Chapter 2, Substance Use Disorder, Codependency, and Family Roles, provides the family member with a relatable understanding of the disease. The video *Pleasure Unwoven* (McCauley 2017) discusses the disease and provides a great explanation of the process of moving from using substances to being addicted to substances. The book *When the Servant Becomes the Master* (Powers 2012) is for the nonexpert and also provides an understandable description of addiction.

- **SUPPORT GROUP MEETINGS.** Hearing other family members talk about their denial of their loved one's SUD does two essential things. First, it allows the family member to hear stories of how others started in denial and then moved from denial to acceptance. Second, it normalizes denial. The family member learns that denial is a normal part of recovery. This normalization makes it easier for the family member to accept their denial.

- **PATIENCE.** Be patient with the family member. Changes in denial start when the family member has built the support system and has the emotional resilience to no longer need the denial defense mechanism. As we all know, this happens, "Sometimes quickly and sometimes slowly."

THE FAMILY MEMBER DENYING THEY NEED HELP

"I do not need help; my loved one does!" More often than not, this statement is the result of not understanding the disease of SUD, how the disease affects the family, and the family's impact on the loved-one's recovery. Resistance to getting help is often further fueled by pride, anger, frustration, shame, fear, guilt, cultural norms, and, sometimes a desire to punish the loved one. Another version of this statement is, "I do not need *your* help!" A family member in early recovery may look at our coaches/counselors and "see" the people who sold their loved one drugs. One family member shared later in recovery that they thought all the parents in the family group were "losers" who had nothing to teach them. It is not unusual for a parent who feels this way to stay in the car while their loved one attends a meeting.

In many respects, denying that they need help is the biggest roadblock to family member recovery because it can stop them from engaging. If a family member denies they need help, usually they are in the precontemplation stage of recovery and either Stage 1 or Stage 2 of their codependency. Here are some things a coach can do to help the family members recognize and accept that they need help.

- DISCUSS THE IMPACT OF FAMILY MEMBER INVOLVEMENT ON THE LOVED ONE. The first benefit of family member involvement is that it increases the chances that the loved one will get and remain sober (Substance Abuse and Mental Health Services Administration 2020). Jeff, a parent in long-term recovery from codependency, said the reason he stayed was that he misheard the person giving the orientation to the program Jeff was attending. The person giving the orientation said there was an 80% *higher* chance of a loved one getting sober with parent involvement. What Jeff heard was, "There was an 80% chance of sobriety with parental involvement." The 80% higher chance of sobriety is a number that we could not validate. SAMHSA and others say family involvement enables the loved one's sobriety but does not quantify the benefit. The critical point is that Jeff stayed because he heard family involvement in recovery helps the loved one.

- FRAME RECOVERY AS PROVIDING A NEW SET OF TOOLS. It is effective to talk about family member recovery in terms of gaining a new set of parenting tools. Family members, especially parents/guardians, initially deal with the addicted loved one by using the same tools their parents/guardians taught them. In general, these tools worked well for the family until the loved one began using substances. Recovery provides a new set of tools. Taking this approach defuses the parent's predisposition to view the recommendation to engage in recovery as a condemnation of their parenting skills. Parents/guardians most certainly have heard this directly or obliquely stated numerous times by their family, friends, and, unfortunately, by pastoral leaders.

- **COMMUNITY EDUCATION.** Parents in Stage 1 or Stage 2 codependency are unlikely to seek help unless the legal system or the schools intervene. Work with community partners and schools to educate the population at large and those that routinely interact with families (e.g., school counselors, physicians, therapists, and religious organizations) on the disease of SUD and where to get help. Providing hope is an integral part of community education. Including personal recovery stories in outreach programs is an effective method to provide hope.

- **FAMILY MEMBER EDUCATION.** Educate the family member on SUD, codependency, and the current dangers of drug use. It is essential to provide family members with an understanding of the stages of SUD and the signs and symptoms of drug use, as well as the signs and symptoms of codependency.[17]

- **ENCOURAGE ATTENDING MEETINGS AND ACTIVITIES.** Being with other family members who have already moved into the action phase of recovery is the best way for a family member to recognize how SUD has affected them. More importantly, the family member can experience the

---

17 The prevalence of fentanyl in current illegal drugs and its potency makes even experimental use potentially deadly. **In the era of fentanyl, the issue is no longer just preventing SUD; it is preventing people from dying from taking just one pill with fentanyl in it.** More information on fentanyl is available at www.songforcharlie.org (Song For Charlie 2023) as well as the Drug Enforcement Agency website entitled Fentanyl Awareness (Drug Enforcement Agency 2023).

unconditional acceptance of this new community and gain hope from the successes that family members often share in meetings.

- **KNOCK ON THE CAR WINDOW.** Sometimes, the family member waiting in the car is just waiting for someone to reach out. Often, the family member in the car does not know there is help for them. Knocking on the car window and introducing yourself and the program will usually result in the family member starting to participate.

- **HAVE PATIENCE.** It is sometimes difficult to watch a frantic family member struggle, knowing that the solution is there for the taking. Have compassion for the family member. It can help if the coach remembers that the family member cannot yet see clearly. The family member will see clearly in God's time, not ours.

Lack of Trust in a Higher Power

The 12-Step approach asks the family member to turn their will and life over to God, which seems like giving up to a family member new to recovery. This is difficult for a family member. What is more difficult, however, especially for parents/guardians, is that the family member is turning their loved one's life over to God. This is a gut-wrenching task that requires a special trust, a deep faith, and an intimate relationship with God that few family members have entering recovery. In many cases, the SUD in the family embitters family members towards God. "How could God let this happen to us?"

Developing a relationship with God that allows turning a family member's will and life and the life of their loved one over to the care of God is a beautiful journey. The following tools are helpful in this process:

- **SUPPORT GROUP MEETINGS AND STEP-WORK.** Hearing other group members' struggles and triumphs in their relationship with their Higher Power provides the grounding and encouragement to embark on the relationship journey. The Steps and hearing their sponsor's story provide a well-proven path to a better relationship with God.

- **PRAYER AND MEDITATION.** Prayer and meditation are integral parts of 12-Step programs. AA Step 11 summarizes the importance of prayer and meditation and the purpose of prayer and meditation: "Sought through prayer and meditation to improve our conscious contact with God as we understood Him, praying only for knowledge of His will for us and the power to carry that out." In other words, Step 11 is developing an intimate relationship with God that fosters the family member's ability to understand His will. This close relationship also provides the trust and courage needed to "let go and let God." Chapter 13, Tools to Help Strengthen a Relationship with God, provides tools that can assist family members in improving their relationship with their Higher Power.

- **ATHEIST.** At first, the 12-Step approach seems impossible for an atheist because choosing to call our Higher Power God is often a major roadblock. Often, stressing that it is a Higher Power of their own choosing can overcome this roadblock. If the atheist wishes, their Higher Power can be the reason, the love of the group, or the universe.

    If this approach is unsuccessful, the coach can refer the family member to atheist or secular 12-Step groups. The group, AA Agnostica, has developed a 12-Step approach specifically for atheists/agnostics (AA Agnostica 2023). The AA Agnostica website summarizes multiple alternative

12 Steps developed by various atheist or agnostic groups (AA Agnostica 2012). These steps replace a Higher Power with the wisdom of the group, the wisdom of the universe, or rational thought. Atheists/agnostics often replace prayer and meditation with just meditation. The atheist/agnostic 12 Steps still have the basics of all 12 Steps—admitting powerlessness, believing a power greater than themselves can help, taking an inventory, removing character defects, making amends, and then the maintenance steps.

SMART (Self-Management and Recovery Training) Recovery® is a secular recovery approach that may appeal to the atheist/agnostic. As it states on its website, SMART Recovery® is "...an evidenced-informed recovery method grounded in rational emotive behavioral therapy, and cognitive behavioral therapy, that supports people with substance dependencies or problem behaviors ..." (SMART Recovery 2024) The approach is built on the premise that the individual has the power to overcome addictions.

False Beliefs

A family member's beliefs determine how the family member will react to an event, how the family member views their loved one, how the family member views themselves, and the family member's level of emotional distress. The antithesis of the three C's of recovery is a good summary of the codependent belief system. In the codependent belief system, the family member believes they caused their loved one's SUD, the family member can control their loved one's SUD, and the family member can cure their loved one's SUD. These family members' beliefs are debilitating for the family member and the loved one. Tools to help change non-recovery beliefs include:

- **EDUCATION.** Knowing recovery beliefs is the first step in changing the family member's belief system. Education provides the "head-understanding" of non-recovery and recovery beliefs.

- **WORKING THE 12 STEPS.** Each of the 12 Steps allows the family member to explore essential recovery beliefs with their sponsor. Working the steps provides knowledge, expands the "head-understanding," and begins the "heart-understanding" of recovery beliefs.

- **SUPPORT GROUP MEETINGS.** Support group meetings provide the "heart-understanding" of recovery beliefs that is the real driver for changing a person's beliefs. Hearing other family members talk about recovery beliefs and their impact on their lives allows the family member to evaluate their beliefs in a non-threatening environment. Hearing stories about how recovery beliefs changed family members' lives gives both the confidence and the courage to change often long-held beliefs.

- **MOVING FROM CODEPENDENT BELIEFS TO RECOVERY BELIEFS TOOL..** Chapter 14, Moving from Non-recovery Beliefs to Recovery Beliefs, uses the event-emotion-belief-feeling-action (EEBFA) model to explain the relationship between an event, what a person believes, and the feeling a person has due to the event. The worksheet with the chapter allows the family member to explore how substituting recovery beliefs for non-recovery beliefs improves his ability to respond to the loved one with kindness and love. As importantly, the family member experiences how adopting recovery beliefs can bring joy back into their life.

Guilt and Shame

Guilt is, "I did something wrong." Shame is, "I am wrong." Guilt and shame are potent recovery inhibitors. Both hinder an intimate relationship with a Higher Power. Both shame and guilt generate unwarranted anger. Both reinforce the belief that the family member deserves the turmoil and anxiety associated with SUD in the family. Most importantly, both shame and guilt hinder or even block the family member's willingness to allow the loved one to feel the consequences of the loved one's substance use. One family member wanted to continually bail her son out because of her perceived shortcomings as a mother. She said, "I owe him because of my failures as a mom. I did not have time for him. Now I need to make up for that."

The most common sources of guilt and shame are the false beliefs engendered by the antithesis to the three C's—cause, cure, and control. Unless you have been there, it is difficult to imagine the level of guilt and shame that you not only caused this fatal disease but also that you have the power to cure it and control your loved one, but you are failing to do so. Think about that last sentence for a couple of minutes. Now imagine that everyone in your family and circle of friends reinforces these false beliefs directly or indirectly.

There is also the guilt/shame a family feels because it is "that family." Most families never wanted to be "that family" with an addict/alcoholic. Many times, other family members criticized and judged "that family." This can be a powerful impediment to recovery primarily because of the isolation and the feeling of unworthiness that slowly permeates each family member. Isolation and unworthiness tend to cause family members to be too ashamed to seek help and believe they are not worthy of help. Tools that help work through guilt and shame include:

- **SUPPORT GROUP MEETINGS.** Just walking into a meeting can be incredibly healing. First, the family member knows that they are not alone. In their community, they might be "that family." In a support group meeting, they are with many other "that families." Second, group meetings teach family members that SUD strikes all types of families. Many family members feel guilty because of divorce. There will be couples in the meeting who have never divorced. Some family members feel guilty because they are poor. People from all socio-economic levels will be at the meeting. Some family members feel guilty over past or current substance abuse. There will also be family members who have never used mind-altering substances. There may be addiction counselors in the same room who understand SUD, but despite the addiction counselor's training, the counselor is at a loss over how to handle their loved one.

- WORKING THE 12 STEPS. Guilt and shame fester in the darkness. Working with a sponsor provides the family member with a safe relationship to bring the shame and the guilt into the light. The inventory (Step 4) and the amends step (Step 9) provide a proven methodology to clear away or at least dampen guilt and shame.

- APPOINTMENTS. Appointments will help with all the roadblocks. Appointments are under guilt and shame because some family members, especially those in Stage 3 and Stage 4 Codependency, believe they do not deserve the recovery coach's time. A coach normalizing the family member's experience, suggesting an appointment, or calling later can reaffirm the family member's worth.

- See Chapter 15, Overcoming Guilt and Shame. This chapter provides tools a recovery coach may use to help a family member work through guilt/shame.

- **AGAPE LOVE THE FAMILY MEMBER.** Like the person with an addiction when she is high, the family member you are working with is under the influence of codependency. Underneath the angry, anxiety-ridden, depressed, sometimes spiteful exterior is a person who dearly loves the loved one who brought them to your door. Fall in agape with the real person in front of you.

- **BE PATIENT WITH THE FAMILY MEMBER'S GUILT OR SHAME.** In many cases, guilt or shame has been festering for so long that it becomes an integral part of the person. The guilt or shame may remain even after the family member realizes the guilt or shame is unfounded or the family member has gone through the amends process. One approach to giving the family member patience is to say what Eric Daxon often says, "My job in removing my character defects or my guilt is to do the work. God removes the character defect or guilt when He no longer needs them to mold me. I do the work. I wait. God removes my defect or my guilt."

Grief

A family member often hides the grief they are feeling. Most family members understand grieving the loss of a loved one to SUD. In general, they do not understand the need to mourn the loss of the things they value. For a parent/guardian, examples of this type of loss include the loss of the dreams they had for their loved one, the loss of the loved one they knew before SUD, and the loss of the relationship they had with their loved one. The family member needs to know that their loved one is also grieving the losses caused by their substance use; surprisingly, recovery also generates a sense of loss that the family member needs to identify and grieve. The same is true when the loved one enters recovery. Tools that aid in dealing with grief include:

- EDUCATION. It is helpful for family members to know that part of what they are experiencing is grief. Knowing that they are grieving and what is causing the grief usually brings relief to the family member. Understanding that their loved one is also grieving fosters empathy for what the loved one is going through.

- SUPPORT GROUP MEETINGS. Hearing other group members talk about their grief and how they deal with it is both validating and helpful.

- SEE CHAPTER 16, RECOGNIZING AND DEALING WITH GRIEF. This chapter discusses the Kubler-Ross stages of grief and provides tools to assist the family member. Chapter 16 also discusses the grief felt by the family member and loved one when they are both in their diseases (codependency and SUD) and when the family member and the loved one are in recovery.

Parting Thoughts on Barriers to Recovery

The barriers listed in this chapter are not the only barriers to family member recovery. Significant gaps in any of SAMHSA's four pillars of recovery (health, home, purpose, and physical needs) are substantial barriers that recovery coaches/counselors need to enable the family member to resolve. The obstacles listed here prevent a family member from working in a personal recovery program based on the 12 Steps. Personal recovery will not solve all of the significant gaps in SAMHSA's four pillars. However, personal recovery will give the family members the tools, mental ability, and emotional strength to develop solutions to their problems. Putting it more succinctly, personal recovery leads to the family member living a self-directed life, which is one of SAMHSA's three objectives for recovery (Substance Abuse and Mental Health Services Administration 2012).

CHAPTER 10

Boundaries for Families Dealing with Substance Use Disorder

A boundary, in its simplest terms, is a demarcation between areas. In recovery, there are multiple areas where boundaries come into play. A personal boundary can be the dividing line between what is acceptable to you and what is not. It can be the line that defines your responsibility and what is not yours. They define who you let in and who you do not. In some instances, boundaries can be flexible. For example, you might not accept a hug from someone when you first meet them. You might agree to the hug after you get to know them better. Cloud and Townsend's book *Boundaries* is an excellent resource for these types of boundaries (Cloud and Townsend 1992).

The boundaries we are discussing here are boundaries are for people dealing with a loved one with SUD. In this chapter, we will discuss two types of boundaries. The first is what the family member will do in response to a loved one doing something objectionable. This is the "If you choose to do this, I will do that" boundary. The second type is those things a family member will not do because they enable the loved one's substance use. A good example is, "I will not lie for you." The objectives of this chapter are to:

- Describe a boundary's purpose.
- Provide methods to help family members identify when they need boundaries.
- Describe the process for a family member to establish good boundaries.
- Explain the motivation for consequences and the process for establishing consequences.

The family member needs to develop these boundaries carefully because, unlike other types of boundaries, they must be enforced each time they are crossed. They are not flexible because they deal with family safety, responding to illegal activity, and not helping a life-threatening disease progress. The family member can change their boundaries through the same deliberate process used to establish them.

The Purpose of a Boundary

The primary purpose of boundaries is to restore sanity to the family by making the 11th Promise of AA a reality for a family member: "We will intuitively know what to do in situations that used to baffle us." Eric talks about the 11th Promise being his favorite from the first time he heard it because, like almost every other family member, he and his wife Joanne had no idea how to respond to their teen's substance use and behavior while using substances. They didn't know what to do when their teen came home high, what to do when the teen ran away or skipped school, or when they found stolen property. Eric and Joanne often argued over what to do next. The arguments were often strident because both, especially Eric, were afraid of what would happen if they did the wrong thing.

Boundaries and the boundary-setting process ameliorated Eric and Joanne's fear and anxiety. Their boundaries resolved the three "what" issues. The first "what" was what behaviors Eric and Joanne would not tolerate. The second "what" was what they were going to do in response to the objectionable behavior. The third "what" was what Eric and Joanne would not do because these actions would enable their teen.

The boundaries themselves were the intellectual or the "head" part of this effort. Eric and Joanne understood what they were going to do. The boundary-setting process provided the confidence, courage, and faith they needed to actually implement the boundaries. In other words, this process provided the "heart." The boundary-setting process gave Joanne and Eric confidence that their response was appropriate because each boundary was discussed with their recovery coach. Understanding that boundaries were put in place to protect Eric and Joanne, their other children, and their loved one gave Eric and Joanne the "heart" they needed to put good boundaries in place and, more importantly, enforce them. Specifically, boundaries are intended to accomplish the following objectives:

- **GIVE THE FAMILY MEMBER AND THE FAMILY THEIR LIVES BACK.** SUD takes an emotional toll on the family member and the family. Arguing over how to respond to the loved one's SUD, strains the relationship between spouses/partners and the rest of the family, often to the point of breaking up the marriage/relationship and the family. Setting and learning to enforce good boundaries eliminates one of the primary sources of emotional discord—what to do when the loved one is in trouble because of SUD. The boundary-setting process is systematic and gives the members of the family confidence that what they are doing is correct, in their best interest, and in the best interest of their loved one.

- **ENSURE THE LOVED ONE FEELS THE NATURAL CONSEQUENCES OF THEIR ACTIONS.** Unfortunately, feeling the pain caused by substance use is one of the prime motivators for a loved one to choose recovery. Boundaries help family members resist the urge to shield their loved one from these consequences. If the loved one is an adult, boundaries aid family members in ensuring the adult loved one bears the total economic and legal burdens of their substance use.

- **PROTECT THE FAMILY MEMBER, THEIR FAMILY, AND THE LOVED ONE.** Boundaries protect the family member and the family from the consequences of the loved one's SUD. Many of the loved one's actions can place the family at risk physically, emotionally, legally, and financially. Boundaries ensure that the family's responses to risky or illegal behaviors mitigate these risks. For example, not allowing a using loved one to drive the family car protects the family from the legal and financial consequences of the loved one being arrested or getting into an accident. More importantly, it also protects the loved one. Getting into an accident and hurting or killing themselves or others will change the loved one's life for the worse. The discussion in the section Using Appendix I: Example Boundaries for Minors and Adults has detailed examples of how boundaries protect the family and the loved one.

- **HELP THE FAMILY NOT ENABLE THE LOVED ONE'S SUBSTANCE USE.** There are overt ways a family member enables a loved one's substance use and ways that are not as obvious. Overt enabling includes giving money, not enforcing boundaries, and allowing using adults to live at home. Getting arrested, getting into accidents, and running out of money can all be due to the loved one's SUD. Bailing the loved one out of jail, paying for the repairs on the car, or giving them money for a "fresh start" all cushion the loved one and prevent them from feeling the adverse consequences that the loved one so desperately needs to choose recovery.

The less overt enablers include yelling, blaming, and shaming the loved one. Demeaning the loved one adds to the shame and guilt they already feel, which is one of the reasons often cited for the loved one's substance use. The loved one does not need an excuse to use, but the longer they have excuses, the longer it is till they realize that the problem is not external but internal. Subtler still, the family member's misery often provides an excuse by allowing the loved one to shift blame to the family.

> Both my children had a real battle with sobriety. There were prolonged periods of sobriety followed by prolonged periods of drug use. The first relapse for each was a time of anger and resentment for me. "How could they do this to me?!!," drove my response. Over time I recognized that they were not doing it to me. They were in the grip of a deadly disease and relapse was one of the symptoms of that disease.
>
> Later in my recovery each of my children crossed major boundaries. I confronted them both with "I" statements that conveyed the love I had for them and the sorrow that I felt enforcing the boundary. There were no arguments and no fighting. I was sad but I was able to go on living a joy filled life. One confrontation occurred on New Year's Eve. My wife and I still went to the PDAP New Year's Eve party and had a wonderful time. The other occurred before a trip we had planned. My wife and I went on the trip. We were sad and worked through the sadness. We had a wonderful time on the trip. As one of the recovery sayings goes, "Sadness is a part of recovery; but misery is optional." By confronting with love, I was choosing sadness and rejecting misery. Anonymous Family Group Member

Key Concepts for Setting and Enforcing Boundaries

In many respects, the boundaries put in place are based on the level of care needed by the loved one and the loved one's actions. Take, for example, the boundary, "If you relapse, you are choosing to either go to residential treatment or not live in our home." Putting this boundary in place at the beginning of a recovery journey is unreasonable because relapse is a part of the disease and will, more than likely, occur several times. Putting a boundary in place about driving for a loved one who does not drive serves no useful purpose. The need to change boundaries as the disease progresses is the reason we recommend that one of the consequences for using is making an appointment with the loved one's recovery coach. The purpose of the appointment is to reexamine the loved one's recovery plan and the family member's boundaries.

The second key concept is that the family member needs to enforce the boundary every time the loved one crosses it. If the family member cannot do this, it is better not to put the boundary in place. Selectively or capriciously enforcing a boundary is a disservice to the loved one and the family. Not enforcing a boundary leads the loved one to believe they can cross it with impunity. If family members enforce boundaries every time the loved one crosses them, the loved one will expect and accept that the family member will consistently enforce their boundaries. Bobby, a family group father, consistently enforced the boundaries on his son. At first, the son tried to escape the consequences by arguing and yelling. Bobby persisted in enforcing the boundaries. Eventually, all Bobby had to say when his son crossed a boundary was, "You know what is coming next?" The son would say, "I know dad." The consistent enforcement of boundaries eventually leads to the loved one coming to accept and expect the consequences.

The third concept is that the family member needs to enforce the boundary from a position of love for the loved one. Enforcement with anger shifts the loved one's focus from what they did to what the family member is doing. Enforcing with anger drains the family member and continues to drain the family member as they relive the encounter. No one wants to be angry with someone they love. Giving the family members other words and tools to enforce a boundary is essential. Statements like, "I love you, and I am sorry things have turned out this way" or "I love you very much, and I just cannot watch you do this to yourself" are effective ways to start enforcing boundaries. Hearing these words increases the likelihood that the family member will use them. It also increases the likelihood that the loved one will focus on what they did and what is happening to them because of what they did. These loving words will not come easily if the family is still struggling with resentment, but there is a higher chance they will come if the family member has already heard them and believes that this is the right approach. Remember, most of the world tells the family to "Come down hard on the loved one!" or "Give them another chance!" Using the ROAD tool discussed in Chapter 10 can assist family members in dealing with resentments that often undergird this type of anger.

Using Appendix F: Do You Need Boundaries in Your Life?

Often, a family member is unaware of the need for boundaries. The progression through the stages of codependency can be gradual enough that the family does not notice the chaos that has crept into their lives. QUESTION 1 of Appendix F: Do You Need Boundaries in Your Life? on page 319, is a list of questions to help the family member see the need for boundaries and identify the main blocks to boundary-setting. You can ask the family members the following questions or ask them to complete the worksheet.

- Are you constantly walking on eggshells?

- Are you worried that you might say or do the wrong thing and not know what the wrong thing is?

- Do you dread going home because you do not know what chaos awaits you and have no idea what to do next? Do you doubly dread the weekends and holidays?

- Are you constantly trying to appease the loved one to the point that you neglect yourself and the rest of your family?

- Do you invoke a consequence, later apologize to your loved one, and rescind the consequence?

- Are you hypervigilant? Are you constantly watching what your loved one does? Do you think about your loved one all the time?

- Do you cover for a loved one (lie for him, call in sick for her, do his homework, bail her out of jail, make excuses to the school for absences or being tardy)?

- Do you go out of your way to please your loved one and avoid conflict?

- Is your loved one always disrespecting you?

- Is your loved one violent in the house, breaking things, punching holes in the walls, threatening, or assaulting people?

- Do you routinely feel resentful toward your loved one?

- Do you routinely feel pushed into doing things you do not want to do, especially with your loved one?

- Do you feel guilty saying "no" even when "no" is the correct answer?

- Do you believe you are responsible for your loved one's happiness?

- Is there a lot of yelling and shouting in your home?

- Does your loved one get what they want by constant badgering?

- Do you constantly find drugs in your house and do nothing for fear of what your loved one will do?

QUESTIONS 2, 3, and 4 ask the family member to identify those causing the most disruption, fear, and resentment in the family member's life. The statements the family member selected give insight into what boundaries the family member needs and also provide insights into the barriers preventing setting and enforcing good boundaries. QUESTION 5, the final question, is, "What would your life be like if none of the above statements were true?" This question aims to generate the hope that a family member needs to decide to set and enforce good boundaries. This is also a suitable time to review the characteristics of SUD, focusing on the need for their loved ones to feel the consequences of their substance use. Going over the three C's can also be beneficial. You did not cause it. You cannot control it. You cannot cure it.

Boundary-Setting Process

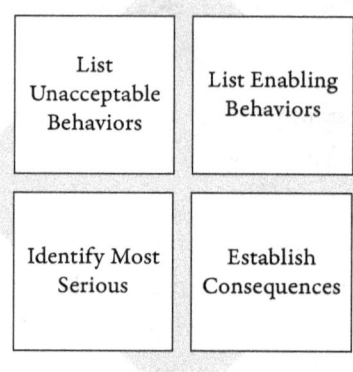

FIGURE 14. APPROACH TO SETTING BOUNDARIES

Once the family member agrees to work on boundaries, *Figure 14* shows the general boundary-setting process. The first difference between the initial and formal boundaries is that the formal process includes identifying the family's actions that enable the loved one to continue using. The second difference is that this process addresses the significant barriers to families setting and enforcing good boundaries and strategies to overcome these blocks. Sometimes, these blocks are so substantial that the family member needs to address them before the boundaries are in place. This section also discusses strategies the recovery coach can use when family members are unwilling to set and enforce good boundaries.

LIST THE LOVED ONE'S UNACCEPTABLE BEHAVIORS

The family member is asked to list everything a loved one does that the family member does not like. This includes substance use-related behaviors (e.g., being high, stealing, lying, dealing, yelling, verbal abuse, etc.) and non-substance use-related behaviors (e.g., dirty room, not doing chores, not doing homework, truancy, loud music, etc.). Encourage the family member to be as thorough as possible. One suggestion is to ask them to answer this question over the period between appointments. This longer observation period usually provides a complete list. Identifying all unacceptable behaviors and not just those related to drug use, accomplishes the following:

- Allows the family member to get it all out on paper. This kind of dumping can bring relief because it sheds light on issues the client may have been hiding.

- Provide the recovery coach with an understanding of what happens in the home with the parent and the loved one.

- Provides insight into the family member's state of mind and areas the recovery coach may need to address in future appointments.

- Identifies all unacceptable behaviors. This will minimize the need to add additional boundaries later.

- Helps to identify the family's unacceptable enabling behaviors.

- Allows the family member to carefully look at each behavior and sift the important from the unimportant. In other words, it allows them to choose the battles they want to fight.

- Allows the family member to identify their part in the family chaos.

- Overcomes many of the roadblocks to setting and enforcing boundaries.

LIST THE FAMILY MEMBER'S ENABLING BEHAVIORS

The family member is asked to identify how they enable their loved one's substance use. This is the first step in developing a different kind of boundary because it is not about what the loved one does. It is a boundary to stop family members from enabling their loved one's substance use. Examples of enabling behaviors are:

- **NOT CONSISTENTLY ENFORCING BOUNDARIES OR NOT ENFORCING THEM AT ALL.** This is one of the most destructive behaviors because the loved one comes to believe that he can manipulate the family member into not enforcing a boundary. Consistently enforcing good boundaries leads the loved one to expect the family member to enforce boundaries. This reduces the stress on both the loved one and the family member. If the family member is not going to enforce a boundary, it is better not to set it.

- **LYING FOR A LOVED ONE.** This includes writing a note when the loved one skips school, calling work and covering for the loved one when they skip work, being dishonest with the police, probation officer, or parole officer when they call, and being dishonest with family members when they ask questions.

- **GIVING A LOVED ONE CASH.** In active addiction, cash will support the loved one's substance use. This includes paying for an adult loved one's housing, food, utility bills, car, car repairs, car insurance, or phone. Money is also a significant trigger for a person with SUD. A family group member once attended a workshop for addicts searching for recovery. The leader asked the group, "What is our biggest trigger?" The instantaneous response from every attendee was "money!"

- **EXPRESS APPROVAL OF ILLEGAL SUBSTANCE USE.** Family members must state their disapproval of illicit substance use, including underage drinking and underage marijuana use in states where marijuana use is legal. This is especially important for underage substance use.

- **USING ILLEGAL DRUGS OR ABUSING ALCOHOL.** The family member using illicit drugs or abusing alcohol can trigger a loved one who is trying to stay sober. In addition, it incentivizes the loved one to use substances.

- **DEMEANING, SHAMING, OR YELLING AT A LOVED ONE.** There are multiple reasons for not demeaning, shaming, or yelling at the loved one. The first is that the loved one with SUD is already feeling guilt and shame whether they show it or not. Adding to the guilt and shame incentivizes use. Second, the loved one is more likely to hear the family member if the family member is speaking from a position of love. Third, it reduces the remorse the family member will feel after enforcing the boundary.

> **WHAT'S IMPORTANT**
>
> "My wife and I let go of two things that were initially high on our priority list. The first was our kids keeping their rooms clean. We realized how unimportant this was when a counselor asked what was more important, 'Them cleaning their rooms or them living.' In discussions with the counselor, we found that we could live with their rooms being messy, but we could not live with their mess in the rest of the house. So, if we found an item of theirs in the rest of the house, we took it to the garage. This worked. Their mess was either in the garage or their room. Our house, not their rooms, stayed clean.
>
> "The second thing was smoking cigarettes. Yes, it did increase the risk later in life, but it was not immediately lethal as were the drugs they were using. Our boundary was we would not buy cigarettes for them.
>
> "Many disagreed with us, but each family is different, and this worked for our family. It relieved one source of stress in the family and gave us the emotional room we needed to restore sanity in other areas of our lives."
>
> ANONYMOUS
> FAMILY GROUP MEMBER

EVALUATE AND SELECT THE MOST SERIOUS BEHAVIORS

The purpose here is to narrow the list of unacceptable behaviors to those that are the most disruptive to the family member and pose a serious safety, financial, or legal risk to the family member. The recovery coach's goal here is to assist the client in identifying which behaviors listed need to be boundaries, which may need to be rules, and which the client will let go of. The recovery coach's task is to help the family member focus on the purpose of setting a boundary. Which objectionable actions become boundaries is the family member's decision. Reviewing the purpose and critical concepts for the boundary-setting process discussed above will aid the family member's winnowing process.

ESTABLISH CONSEQUENCES

The consequences are actions the family member will take in response to the loved one crossing a boundary. There are a couple of guidelines when selecting consequences:

- **CONSEQUENCES NEED TO PROMOTE THE OBJECTIVES OF SETTING BOUNDARIES.** For example, if a loved one is using substances, they cannot drive the car. A parent allowing a using loved one to drive the parent's car places them, the loved one, and others at risk. Getting into an accident can seriously harm the loved one or others. This also puts the family at financial risk—letting someone drive that the family member knew was using is contributory negligence if the loved one is in an accident. This can and has resulted in the injured party suing the family for damages.

- **CONSEQUENCES ARE NOT PUNISHMENTS.** The intent of a consequence is not to punish but to protect the loved one and the family and not enable the loved one's use of drugs. Understanding this helps the family member enforce a boundary with love rather than anger.

- **CONSEQUENCES ARE NOT INTENDED TO GET THE LOVED ONE TO STOP USING SUBSTANCES.** It is common for family members to say the boundaries are not working because their loved one is still using substances. If this is the case, remind the family member that the purpose of boundaries is to protect the family member, protect the family, protect the loved one, not enable the loved one's drug use, and give the family member his life back. If there are good boundaries and the family member is enforcing them, they are working because the family is ensuring safety and not helping their loved one use.

- **THE CONSEQUENCES ARE, TO AS GREAT AN EXTENT AS POSSIBLE, THE NATURAL OUTCOMES OF THE ACT.** Sometimes, the family does not need to do anything except let the natural outcome occur. For example, if the loved one does not do their homework, they will get a zero. Enough zeros, and they will fail. If they are driving under the influence and a police officer pulls them over, they will get a citation, and the police officer may arrest them. The family's role is to allow these consequences and not soften the blow.

- **THE CONSEQUENCES OFFER HOPE OF RESTITUTION.** Where possible, there should be a sobriety-related time limit for the consequence. For example, a loved one uses, and they cannot use the family car until they are 30 days sober. Putting a definite length of time lets the loved one know the consequence is not forever and gives them a solid, sobriety-related target to shoot for. Setting an ambiguous period like "when I think you are ready" is more of an effort to control the loved one. That is not the purpose of a boundary. The ambiguous consequence also allows for abuse both by the family member enforcing the boundary and the loved one. The main reason for setting a specific period is to reduce the potential for the loved one's manipulation to be successful. The length of time is no longer up to the discretion of the family member.

Using Appendix G: Identify the Loved One's Unacceptable Behaviors and Family Member Enabling Behaviors

Appendix G provides a worksheet for the family member to identify the loved one's unacceptable behaviors and the family member's enabling behaviors. Worksheet QUESTION 1, on page 321, asks the family member to list all of the loved ones objectionable behaviors. Those related to substance use as well as those that are not.

QUESTION 2 starts the winnowing process for the family member by asking the family member to identify those behaviors that cause the most disruption in the family member's life and the most disruption to the whole family. This is the beginning of identifying the behaviors that warrant establishing boundaries. The essential parts of QUESTION 2 are the sub-bullets a through c. These ask the family member to describe the impact their loved one's behavior had on the family member, their significant other, and the rest of the family. It is essential to ensure that the family member's answers are thorough, so the family member understands the full impact of the loved one's behavior.

QUESTION 3 asks the family member what they have done in response to the loved one's unacceptable behaviors and whether this has worked. Yelling and shouting are common responses. Demeaning and shaming are counterproductive to recovery and usually do not change the loved one's behavior. Rather than pointing out that the parenting tool of raising their voice did not work for a loved one with SUD, it is better to allow the family member to say it. Framing the boundary-setting process as providing the family member with another tool specifically designed for dealing with loved ones with SUD acknowledges that the family member did what they knew how to do. The family member was not wrong. The family member needed another tool in his toolbox.

It is important to understand that family members respond to their loved ones with the tools they have. Yelling to induce guilt and shame can effectively correct children's and teens' behavior. These are not optimal by today's standards, but they do work. Eric and Joanne had five children. Before SUD entered their family, both used raised voices (yelling) and punishment (grounding) to correct their children's behavior. These worked until SUD took two of their children. Of course, Eric and Joanne continued using the tools they knew and had previously worked for them. They continued until they understood SUD, codependency, and recovery. They continued using their old tools until they added boundaries to their toolbox. From then on, boundaries and the boundary process were how they responded to their loved one's unacceptable behavior. It is important not to condemn family members directly or indirectly for responding to their loved ones with the only available tools.

This is another excellent opportunity to discuss what the family member can and cannot control. This is also an ideal place to reinforce the concept that a boundary's purpose is to give the family their lives back, protect the family (including the loved one), and not enable the loved one's substance use.

QUESTION 4 in Appendix G asks the family member to list their enabling behaviors. QUESTION 4A and QUESTION 4B address what the loved one and the family member get from these enabling behaviors. What the loved one gets from the enabling behavior is obvious: the ability to continue using substances with no or minimal consequences. The family member benefits are not as obvious but just as real. First, they do not have to feel fear of anticipating the blowback of enforcing a boundary. The loved one's blowback can be just spiteful words, destroying property, physical violence, or running away. The flipside to not implementing or sporadically enforcing boundaries is that the family member can be the "good guy." One father said, "I wanted to see my son smile at me."

Using Appendix H: Boundary-Setting Handout

Appendix H: Boundary-Setting Handout on page 323 can assist the family members in developing their boundaries. Appendix I: Example Boundaries for Minors and Adults has example boundaries that the recovery coach can use if the family member gets stuck or if the family member needs to revise the boundary to be in line with the objectives of setting boundaries. The worksheet has questions designed to encourage the family member to think about what life is like currently and what life would be like if the boundary were in place.

QUESTION 1 in the boundary-setting handout asks the family member to identify the most serious unacceptable behaviors they have listed in Appendix G: Identify the Loved One's Unacceptable Behaviors. They are asked to list at least three and no more than ten. The reason for the limits is to push those family members that tend to minimize and restrain those that are over zealous. There may end up being more or less, and that is okay. The recovery coach's role here is to assist the family member in choosing behaviors that jeopardize the family member, the rest of the family, and the loved one. Reminding the family member of a boundary's objectives assists in this process.

QUESTION 2 identifies the consequence if the loved one crosses the boundary and asks the family member to write the boundary in the format, "If you (unacceptable action), I will (consequence)." The consequences need to meet the criteria for consequences already discussed.

It is important to note that the boundary does not start by telling the loved one what not to do. It begins by stating what the unacceptable is and what the family member will do in response. The boundary concerning violence does not start with, "Do not be violent…" The boundary begins with, "If you are violent, I will call the police." The reason for the difference is threefold. First, telling someone not to do something often encourages them to do it. Second, it reinforces the concept that the family member cannot control what the loved one chooses to do. The family member can only control their actions. Third, and more importantly, simply stating the objectionable behavior without favor or disfavor places the decision to do the objectionable behavior squarely and solely on the loved one. The loved one has the power of choice. This boundary construct respects the loved ones' right to choose. It also respects the family member's right to decide what to do in response to the loved one's choice.

QUESTION 3A asks the family member to think about what they gain by not setting the boundary. This may seem counterintuitive, but it is not. By not setting the boundary, the family member can:

- **AVOID AN ANGRY CONFRONTATION WITH THE LOVED ONE.** No one enjoys having a boundary set on them. In most families, boundaries change the family homeostasis. The loved one will suffer consequences that are not in place before boundaries.

- MAINTAIN THE *STATUS QUO*. There is a great deal of comfort in leaving things as they are. Depending on the family member's stage of codependency, the family member might be quite comfortable in a chaotic environment because the family member gets accustomed to the chaos.

- AVOID "RUINING" THEIR LOVED ONE'S LIFE. Many consequences involve calling the police, reporting the loved one truant, not bailing the loved one out, or not doing the loved one's homework. Part of the anxiety associated with ruining a loved one's life is related to the family member's love for the loved one. However, part of the problem is the family member's concern for themselves. The family member hates the thought of what a loved one ruining their own life will do to the family member. This is a self-centered and selfish reason for the family member not setting and enforcing boundaries. The recovery coach must point out this self-centeredness and selfishness lovingly and at the right time.

- REMAIN THE "HERO." Boundaries require letting go. Many family members do not want to let go early in recovery because they still believe they can save their loved one, and *they want the credit for doing so*. Rick said, "I wanted to be the one that saved my daughter. I knew I would find the words that would get her to 'see the light.' I imagined her saying to me years later, 'Dad, remember when you said….' that is what got me sober." Be patient with these family members. Pride is a character defect that God can and will remove when the time is right.

- BE THE "NICE" PARENT/GUARDIAN. Parents/guardians want their children to like them. Wanting to be liked is a powerful motivator. Rick said, "I just wanted my son to smile at me." Family members often believe that the loved one will love/like them more if the family member does not set and consistently enforce good boundaries. Usually, the opposite occurs; the loved one resents the non-boundary-enforcing family member, especially when the loved one is in recovery. As Eric Daxon says, "I have never heard an addict say they got sober because their parents were nice to them."

QUESTION 3B asks the family member what they gain by setting a boundary. These will be different for each family member. Here are some suggested benefits if the family member is stuck:

- KNOWING WHAT TO DO IN SITUATIONS THAT USED TO "BAFFLE" THE FAMILY MEMBER. This is the most crucial benefit of boundaries. Much of the anxiety and turmoil in the family comes from wrestling with how to respond to a loved one's acting out. Once the boundaries are set, the family member and the loved one know the consequences. The boundary-setting process provides the confidence that the boundary is sound and that the consequence is appropriate and kind.

- PERSONAL SAFETY AND SAFETY FOR THE FAMILY. A boundary does not prevent the loved one from harming the family because it is enforced after the loved one acts out. A good boundary dissuades the loved one from acting out because they know the consequences. If written correctly, a good boundary also adds to familial safety by encouraging the family to act before the violence escalates. Often, a family member will not respond to a loved one's violence until the violence results in severe injury. A good boundary will encourage action as soon as the violence starts. An effective way to explain this is to ask the family member, "Do you want your loved one arrested for simple assault, assault, aggravated assault, manslaughter, or murder?" Like SUD, family violence usually escalates as the disease worsens.

QUESTION 3C asks the family member what the loved one will gain if the family member does not set and enforce boundaries. If boundaries are not set and enforced, the loved one:

- **CAN CONTINUE THEIR SUBSTANCE USE.** This falls under the rubric: "If nothing changes, nothing changes." If the familial environment remains the same, the loved one's behavior will remain the same.

- **RETAINS ONE OF THEIR REASONS FOR USING.** The contradictory thing about codependency is that it encourages the substance-using behavior that the codependent wants so desperately to stop. As already discussed in Chapter 2, Substance Use Disorder, Codependency, and Family Roles, the loved one is already feeling shame and guilt over their addiction. The constant lecturing, anger, shaming, martyr behavior, and hypervigilance associated with codependency exacerbate the loved one's self-hatred and desire to alleviate this feeling through substance use.

QUESTION 3D asks the family member to write down what their loved one will gain if the family member sets and enforces good boundaries. This question may stump a family member, especially if the family member is in early recovery. Here are a couple of examples that may help a family member get un-stumped:

- **RAISES THE LOVED ONE'S "BOTTOM."** Debra Jay, in the book *No More Letting Go: The Spirituality of Taking Action Against Alcoholism and Drug Addiction,* makes two critical points (Jay 2006). First, a person with SUD does not need to hit "rock bottom" to want to get into recovery. "Rock bottom" is defined as experiencing consequences that are so terrible (e.g., divorce, poverty, homelessness, prison, losing children, severe injury, etc.) that the loved one no longer wants to use. Second, the family can take actions that will aid the loved one in choosing recovery before these catastrophic events occur. One of the most essential actions is setting and enforcing good boundaries.

- **ENSURES A CLEAR UNDERSTANDING OF WHAT IS UNACCEPTABLE AND THE CONSEQUENCES OF CROSSING A BOUNDARY.** As odd as it may seem, there is often a lack of understanding of what is acceptable and what is not. If there is no response from the family member to the loved one using illegal drugs, the loved one can assume that the family member allows illicit drug use. This clarity also protects the loved one from the family arbitrarily ratcheting up the consequences when the family member is angry. One of the worst examples occurred when a loved one called his mom at 7 PM to tell her he would be home before curfew (8 PM). He was 45 minutes away. The mom was angry and changed the curfew to 7:30 PM.

- **A FAMILY THAT IS NO LONGER IN CATASTROPHIC DISTRESS.** A family with family members in Stage 3 or Stage 4 Codependency is chaotic. This is a case where both the boundary-setting process and the boundaries themselves reduce the anxiety and fear that fuels Stage 3 and Stage 4 Codependency. The boundary-setting process allowed the family member to examine each of the loved one's stress-inducing behaviors and sift the important from the unimportant. In Joanne and Eric's case, they were no longer stressed over their child's dirty room. They determined, with their counselor, that a messy room was not significant compared to recovery from a life-threatening disease.

Similarly to QUESTION 1, QUESTION 4 asks the family member to review their list of enabling behaviors and select the ones they wish to address. These are behaviors that enable their loved one's substance use. QUESTION 5 asks the family member to write the boundary and like QUESTION 3, QUESTION 6 asks what the family member and the loved one will gain if the boundary is not set and the boundary is put in place. The gains for each are similar to the gains already discussed.

Using Appendix I: Example Boundaries for Minors and Adults

Appendix I: Example Boundaries for Minors and Adults lists recommended boundaries for adult and minor loved ones. The discussion below explains the rationale behind each of the boundaries and the rationale for each of the consequences. Included in this list are boundaries for abusive phone calls or texts from the loved one. It is important to reinforce that setting and enforcing a good boundary is the kindest, most loving thing a family member can do for their loved one.

BEING HIGH OR UNDER THE INFLUENCE

The first boundary in the worksheet has actions a family member can consider taking if they believe the loved one is high. The first point is the boundary states, "If *we believe* (italics added) you are high,.." The boundary does not say,

"If *you are high*,..." This is written this way for two reasons. First, it minimizes the potential argument with the loved one over whether the loved one is high. In general, family members know when their loved one is high. Second, some family members want to be "100% certain" the loved one is using before enforcing a boundary. The 100% sure standard leaves a lot of room for manipulation by the loved one. Saying "believe" clarifies that 100% certainty is not required.

The first consequence for being high is making a counseling/coaching appointment to reevaluate the loved one's recovery plan and the family member's boundaries. This consequence recognizes that SUD is a disease and relapse is a part of SUD. As with any disease, a relapse does not mean you give up. Cancer can be a recurring disease. If one treatment does not work, you try another. If the cancer is gone and then returns, you reevaluate the treatment options and choose the next right choice. The same is true for SUD. If the loved one is high, that means it is time to reevaluate the current recovery plan. The new recovery plan could include intensive outpatient care, partial hospitalization, or inpatient residential treatment.

The second consequence is specifically for an adult loved one because it includes moving out of the home as a consequence. If the family member wants to allow the loved one to return home at a later date, it is important to include the requirements for returning home. Example requirements listed in the appendix include being sober for a certain number of days, completing outpatient treatment, completing inpatient treatment, and completing aftercare requirements.

The third consequence is not allowing the loved one to drive the car until the loved one is at least 30 days sober. This is a safety and financial protection boundary that parents/guardians can set if they own the car and/or provide car insurance. This is an essential boundary because driving under the influence significantly increases the risk of having a serious accident that could injure or kill the loved one, other persons in the car, and others on the road. Allowing the loved one to drive the car when the family member knows the loved one was using or in possession of mind-changing substances places the family at criminal and civil legal risk.

It is important to note that the consequence has an expiration date that is based on sobriety. Before allowing the use of your car or a car you insure, the loved one needs to be sober for at least 30 consecutive days. Remember, it can take several months for someone with SUD to get 30 straight days of sobriety. We recommend no more than 90 days. For a teen, 90 days is an eternity. The family member can increase the length of sobriety required for successive relapses or allow the length to remain the same. If the loved one owns the car and pays their own insurance, this is not a consequence the family member can impose.

The fourth consequence is denying the use of a phone the family pays for. This is a valid consequence if the loved one used the phone to procure the substances or for other illegal purposes. If the loved one paid for the phone and is paying for the service, there is nothing the family member can do. If the family member owns the phone or pays for the service, then the family member can deny phone use.

The family member must understand that the reason for doing this is not to prevent the loved one from making phone calls. More than likely, the loved one will gain access to another phone. The reason for denying the loved one access to a family member-provided phone is for the family member to stop enabling substance use. If the loved one buys their own phone and pays for their own service, that is money they can no longer use to purchase substances. The length of time sober depends on what the family members can enforce and what they believe is reasonable. It is common for a family member to complain that the loved one found another way to get a phone. This is an appropriate time to remind them that the purpose of a boundary is not to get the loved one to stop making drug-related phone calls. The purpose of a boundary is for the family member not to help or enable the loved one to make these calls.

The fifth is only for adults. A family member setting a boundary with the consequence of asking the loved one to leave is difficult. This consequence needs to be put in place after a considerable amount of thought and prayer by the family member. This is a consequence that applies only to adult loved ones with the ability to live alone (not disabled). This boundary is put in place to protect the family and not enable the loved one's substance use. If an adult loved one is living in your home, you are enabling their drug use by providing food and shelter. Even if they are paying rent, the rent they are paying is usually well below market value.

A second reason, you do not need chaos in your life. As one parent put it, "I could not watch my daughter kill herself anymore. It was too painful." This is usually a boundary that the family sets after being in recovery for a while. This is the case for a couple of reasons. First, the family member must have the recovery and the emotional resilience to enforce the boundary. Second, SUD is a relapsing disease, and the loved one needs time to build the recovery program that leads to long-term sobriety.

FINDING SUBSTANCES OR PARAPHERNALIA

The first consequence for finding substances or paraphernalia on your property (e.g., car, home, land you own) is to either throw it away or call the police. We have had mixed results when calling the police. In some instances, the police arrest the loved one, or they give the loved one a warning. Even if the police found substances/paraphernalia in the loved one's room, they may choose to do nothing to the loved one because the whole family had access to the loved one's room. In general, most family members will opt to throw the articles away. The calculus changes if the family member finds substantial quantities. In this instance, we recommend the family member call a recovery coach to discuss options.

Finding substances and paraphernalia is treated the same as if the loved one used substances. Why else would they have it? This also warrants an appointment with coaches/counselors to reevaluate the recovery plan and restricted car use. If the loved one used the phone to purchase the drugs/paraphernalia, then the family member should implement any boundaries they have related to phone use and substances.

RUNNING AWAY OR GOING OUT WITHOUT PERMISSION

The suggested boundary for a minor loved one running away or going out without permission is for the family member to call the police and list the loved one as a runaway. Listing the loved one as a runaway protects the loved one and the family. If the loved one runs away or leaves without permission, what they are doing is likely illegal or unsafe. This boundary protects the loved one in two ways. First, if the police interact with the loved one, the police are more likely to bring the loved one home. Second, listing a minor loved one as a runaway dissuades other families, friends, and people with ill intentions from harboring the loved one. This protects the family member and the family because it documents awareness that the loved one was missing, and it documents that the family member took prudent actions to ensure the loved one's safety.

Encourage the family member to let the police know about the loved one's substance use and any other dangerous behavior the loved one has done in the past. Telling the police about past behaviors provides the information the police need to make an accurate risk assessment and take appropriate actions. Also, if the family member knows where the loved one might have gone, encourage the family member to provide this information to the police. If the family member believes the loved one is in immediate danger, it is essential to relay this information to the police. Often, a family member hesitates to provide this information for fear of being wrong.

Encourage the family member to relay the information even if the family member is not sure. A mom's story illustrates how important this can be. A mom could locate her minor daughter using the daughter's phone. The daughter was at a motel. The mom and her husband learned from the motel clerk that the daughter was in a room with an adult male. The mom called the police and could direct the police to the room. The police found drugs and evidence of human trafficking. The police arrested the man, and the daughter was rescued.

TRUANCY OR SKIPPING CLASSES

There are natural consequences for a loved one being truant or skipping classes. If a loved one does it enough, they will fail. If the parent/guardian knows the loved one is truant, the consequence is that the parent/guardian will call the school and report the absence as unexcused. The family member can add other consequences depending on the circumstances. For example, if the loved one is truant because they were up until 3 AM on their phone and could not get up in time for school, the parent/guardian could deny the loved one using the phone for a specific length of time. The period of time could be just several days (e.g., losing phone privileges for seven days) or the number of days the loved one goes to school. "The phone will be returned after you have gone to school, on time for seven straight days." The advantage of linking the return of phone privileges to attendance is that it enables school attendance. The disadvantage is that the parent/guardian must know if the loved one attended school.

The recommended method for a parent/guardian to determine attendance is to assume the loved one went to school unless the parent/guardian knows differently. The parent/guardian will know if the loved one is truant or late if the loved one does not leave the home in time to be on time. The parent/guardian will also know if the school notifies them. As already discussed, the loved one may find a way to hide truancy. Again, the purpose of the boundary is not to ensure attendance but for the parent/guardian to enable attendance and discourage truancy.

It is common for parents/guardians to place graduating ahead of needed treatment for the loved one. If you have never been a parent/guardian, delaying needed treatment so a loved one can graduate might seem unfathomable. It is important to understand and be compassionate about the real turmoil, shame, and anxiety a parent/guardian can feel because of the prospect of their loved one failing a grade or not graduating from high school. Family members and friends who do not understand SUD can exacerbate this anxiety by providing well-meaning advice on how to get the loved one through high school. Overcoming the parents'/guardians' overwhelming urge to have their loved one graduate is an often slow process that should include education, attending support group meetings, and a hefty dose of compassion from their coach.

ILLEGAL ACTIVITY AND STEALING

Illegal activity is a catch-all boundary for several unacceptable behaviors. The family member may lump illegal behaviors in one boundary as they are in Appendix I: Example Boundaries for Minors and Adults, or the family member can put them in place separately. Notice that there is a separate boundary for stealing. It is important not to "pile on" with this boundary and only put boundaries needed for the specific loved one in place. If the loved one has never been violent, there may be no need for a boundary concerning assault. That does not mean the boundary cannot be put in place later. Whether the boundary is in place or not, the family member can and should call the police if the loved one assaults a family member. The consequence of the illegal behavior in the example boundary is calling the police to report it and then, if appropriate, pressing charges. This is a difficult boundary to enforce because of the potential ramifications of police involvement—arrest, jail, charged with a felony, and prison.

Calling the police is highly recommended if the loved one is violent, threatening violence, or is mentally unstable. This protects the family member from unacceptable behavior. It protects the loved one because the sooner they feel the consequences of violent behavior, the more likely they are to stop. It is better to have the loved one arrested for assault than aggravated assault, manslaughter, or worse.

DISRESPECTFUL BEHAVIOR

A boundary for disrespectful behavior can be as simple as, "If you are disrespectful, I will ask you to stop. If you do not stop, I will walk away." The first part of the boundary asks them to stop because, in some instances, the loved one does not know they are being disrespectful. (Most of us have had children accuse us of yelling and responded, "No. I am not!") Unbelievably, walking away is often remarkably effective. This boundary protects the family member from verbal abuse. Walking away also protects the loved one and the family member because it minimizes the chance of escalating the interaction. The first time a family member enforces this boundary, the loved one may follow the family member.

A second highly effective approach for the family member is to follow the basic rules for fair fighting and use Dick Shaefer's "ignoring skills" found in his book *Choices and Consequences: What to Do When a Teenager Uses Alcohol/Drugs* (Shaefer 1998). First, try not to engage when angry or the loved one is high. Set a time to talk later when the family member is not angry, or the loved one is not under the influence. Second, talk about the present and not the past. Say, "You are lying." Do not say, "You always lie." Third, talk about just the facts. Say, "You punched a hole in the wall." Do not say, "I cannot believe you are destroying our house." Say, "You are acting high." Do not say, "You used drugs again tonight." The family member can say the loved one used substances if the family member saw the loved one use. Fourth, the family member should keep their responses brief.

Do not underestimate the impact of verbal attacks. It is common for the loved one's verbal aggression to turn into physical altercations that result in both physical and emotional damage to the family. In one instance, a family member recorded her child's two-hour rant. In another example, a parent had to get a hotel room for a respite from her son's verbal assaults.

This boundary recognizes that a family member cannot control what the loved one says, but the family member can choose whether they are going to listen.

DAMAGE TO HOME OR PROPERTY

The primary consequence is that the loved one will either repair the damage or will pay to have the damage repaired. It is common for a loved one to refuse to do either. In this case, the parents/guardians have options depending on whether the loved one is a minor or an adult. Here are some options:

- If the loved one is a minor and the parents/guardians have access to their bank accounts, they can pay for the repairs from the minor's account.

- If the loved one is a minor or an adult, parents/guardians can use any funds set aside for their loved one. This includes college funds or, if cash is usually given for special events (birthdays, graduations), the cash can be used to pay for the event. One couple usually bought their children a car for their 16th birthday. They used the money set aside for the vehicle to repair their home.

- If the loved one is an adult and refuses to fix the damage, the parents/guardians can make repairing the damage a condition of continuing to live in the parent's/guardian's home. If the loved one refuses to leave, the family member can evict an adult loved one based on the eviction laws in their state.

SPECIFIC BOUNDARIES FOR AN ADULT LOVED ONE LIVING AT HOME

Many households allow their adult children to remain home if they are full-time students passing their classes or agree to pay rent. The boundaries in this section apply specifically to adults. The family member can change any of the conditions. For example, the condition could be failing no more than one class instead of passing all classes. Instead of two months' rent in arrears, it could be three months in arrears. In addition to protecting the family, these boundaries enable adult behavior in the loved one. Adding the requirement that the full-time student be passing requires the loved one to have the ability to concentrate and requires them to attend class. For the non-students, adding the rent stipulation requires them to get a job and retain enough money to pay the rent.

Notice that all these requirements are outcomes and not process requirements. Process requirements for the full-time student could be doing all their homework on time or attending all their classes. These process requirements would mean the parents/guardians must monitor all homework and attendance. This turns the parents/guardians into helicopter parents who must watch the loved one's day-to-day activities. Setting passing as the standard means the parents/guardians must monitor only at report card time.

A process requirement would require the non-student to have a job to live at home. Requiring a job has several pitfalls. First, it is easy to lie about having a job or lie about looking for employment. In one case, a loved one was routinely applying for jobs but was never hired because the loved one always failed the required drug tests. The loved one told the parents that he did not get the job. Second, a family member can evict a loved one for not paying rent; but the loved one cannot be evicted for not having a job. Like the case with the full-time student, the parents/guardians need to engage on this boundary only once a month instead of constantly asking, "Do you have a job?" The other positive about paying rent versus requiring employment is that paying rent reduces the funds the loved one has available for substance use.

BOUNDARIES FOR PHONE CALLS

Often, loved ones use texts and phone calls to manipulate and act out. This is disruptive and often difficult to live with. The example boundaries for phone calls in Appendix I: Example Boundaries for Minors and Adults are boundaries family members have put in place to protect themselves from manipulation and badgering.

Using Abusive Language

The first phone call boundary deals with abusive language in a phone call, text, or email. The consequence is that the family member will not "listen" to the abuse by hanging up or not answering the text or the email. Like walking away when someone is verbally abusive in person, the family member cannot control what the loved one says or writes, but they can choose not to listen or not respond. The next time it occurs, the family member could leave the blocked time the same or write the boundary to increase the blocked time.

Badgering and Manipulation

The second boundary deals explicitly with a loved one badgering a family member to change a "no" into a "yes." In one case, a mom received 15 texts asking for what the mom had already denied. The texts came while the mom was in a work meeting, and the mom's phone buzzing with each text distracted the mom and others. The mom did not want to turn her phone off because she expected business and meeting-related calls. Blocking the loved one's number and email protected the mom while not interfering with the mom's work.

Harassing Texts or Phone Calls

The third boundary is related to the second and could be combined with the second. It is written as a separate boundary so the family member can make sure the loved one understands that both behaviors—trying to change a yes to a no and trying to harass—are unacceptable. Notice that this boundary does not state a reason for the call. The family member is setting this boundary because the loved one is not respecting the family member's decision not to answer the call or reply to the text immediately.

Hurtful Conversations

The fourth boundary is hanging up when the loved one starts complaining about something in the loved one's power to fix, but the loved one chooses not to fix it. This boundary was put in place by a family member with an alcoholic daughter. The daughter had multiple alcohol-related and non-alcohol-related medical issues, some of which were serious. She would call her mom and complain, but the daughter refused to take the necessary actions to address these issues. These calls saddened, frightened, and depressed the mom. Not talking to her sick daughter was both kind and loving. As long as the mom listened, she was enabling her daughter to stay sick because the daughter had an outlet for her pain. When the mom stopped listening, the mom was no longer enabling her daughter's refusal to seek the medical care the daughter needed.

Threats of Suicide

The fifth phone call boundary is essential. When a loved one talks about suicide in a credible manner, action is required. Calling the mental health unit of the police department ensured that trained officers would respond to the request for a wellness check. Some cities have police officers trained to respond to a mental health crisis. The advantage of having a police officer respond is that they can detain (arrest) and transport the person to a mental health facility without the person's permission. Each municipality has its own criteria for when a police officer can arrest a person for mental health issues. Usually, the requirements include the person must present a danger to themselves or others.

Too Many Phone Calls

The wording of the sixth boundary starts with "I would love to talk to you twice a day..." This makes it clear that the family member wants to talk to the loved one but does not want to be inundated with phone calls.

The major hindrance to blocking a loved one's phone is that the family member wants to be there for the loved one in an emergency. What often helps overcome this hesitancy is reminding the family member that if it is a real emergency, the loved one should call the police, the fire department, or the hospital.

BOUNDARIES TO PREVENT FAMILY MEMBERS FROM ENABLING

The following are examples of boundaries for not enabling the loved one. This type of boundary does not follow the format of "if you do this, I will do this." This boundary is just a statement of what the family member will or will not do for the loved one. Here are some examples:

Do not Give Cash

Giving cash to a loved one in active SUD is, in essence, supporting substance use. Cash is the preferred method for purchasing substances because its value is known, and it is easy to carry out further transactions like the dealer purchasing more substances from his supplier. Giving a gift card for special occasions or necessities (like school lunches) is better because using these in illegal transactions is more complicated. Some parents/guardians gave their loved ones cash cards with accounts that the parents/guardians could monitor. If the parents/guardians suspected illicit activity, they took the card back. These are not foolproof. As one parent stated, "When we gave our Jeanette gift cards, she would sell them at a discount for cash."

Do not Financially Support an Adult Loved One Except for Treatment

This boundary recognizes that SUD is a disease where feeling the consequences of substance use is part of the treatment. The first part of this boundary is feeling the consequences of substance use—financial insecurity or ruin. The second part of the boundary (except for treatment) is recognizing the true nature of SUD; it is a disease. Allowing the loved one to feel the financial consequences includes not providing housing, not cosigning for loans, not providing food, not paying bail, not paying for auto repairs, etc. This is a problematic boundary for a family member to enforce because it can be heartbreaking to think of a loved one being homeless or remaining in jail.

The difficulty and heartbreak are worsened if the adult loved one has children living with them. There are no cut-and-dried solutions to keeping grandchildren safe and not enabling the adult loved one. Give the family members options and help them come to the solution that works for the family member and the family as a whole. Options could include directly paying for housing, food, and utilities, calling child protective services, and seeking custody of the children. Again, there are no simple solutions.

Do not Lie for the Loved One

Lying to protect a loved one shields them from the natural consequences of drug use or alcohol abuse. Telling the truth seems easy, but this can be difficult for a family member. It is hard for a parent to refuse to write an excused absence note for a loved one when one more unexcused absence means the loved one will not graduate high school. It is hard for a parent to lie to a parole officer when telling the truth means their loved one returns to prison. It is hard for a wife to lie to the boss when telling the truth means her husband loses his job. Telling the truth in these difficult situations is easier if the family member understands the disease and has a support system that can cushion the harm to the family member from truth-telling.

Do not Condone the Loved One's Substance Use

This boundary seems obvious, but it is not. Many believe that the loved one can use substances as long as it is not their substance of choice. If this were true, an alcoholic could smoke marijuana or use other mind-altering substances normally. This is not the case. The family needs to make clear that they will not condone the loved one's use of any mind-altering substances.

Do not Use Illegal Substances or Abuse Legal Substances

A family member using illegal substances or abusing legal substances enables the loved one's substance use, particularly if the loved one is living in the same house. First, family use provides access to substances. Some families try placing their substances in locked cabinets, but a loved one in active addiction or a loved one in early sobriety will find a way to gain access. Second, being around people who are using is a strong trigger for a loved one with SUD. This is especially true for loved ones in early recovery.

This creates a dilemma for family members who want to drink alcohol or use marijuana legally. Most family members can abstain until either the loved one is in long-term sobriety or the loved one moves out. There are options if a family member cannot or does not want to abstain. If the loved one is an adult, they can move out or into a sober home. Things are more complicated if the loved one is a minor. A family member's unwillingness to abstain can be due to several issues, such as:

- Not understanding the nature of the disease. Many family members do not understand the progressive nature of the disease and believe the loved one can abstain through willpower.

- Harboring serious resentments towards the loved one. The family turmoil, heartache, and pain from the loved one's SUD is real and often comes out as anger towards the loved one. The family member is unwilling to sacrifice for someone they believe caused the family so much pain.

- Having a substance use issue. Many times, the family member is unwilling to abstain because they have SUD.

Putting Boundaries in Place

Generally, it is up to the person setting the boundaries to determine how and when they will put them in place. The recommended method, especially for minors, is giving the boundaries to loved one in a joint appointment. The substance user, the substance user's coach, the parent/guardian, and their coach are in the appointment. The general flow of the meeting starts with one of the coaches going over what a boundary is and is not. The recovery coach or family member reads the boundaries, and there is an opportunity to ask questions.

The reason for having everyone in the same room is that everyone hears the same thing when the boundaries are established, and any questions can be answered with the group present. This reduces ambiguity and allows each coach to hold all parties accountable for accurately enforcing the boundaries.

Parting Thoughts on Boundaries

The following are general comments related to boundaries:

- **GIVE THE RECOVERY PROCESS A CHANCE TO WORK.** This is important for both the loved one and the family member. Loved ones do not get sober after one meeting or one appointment. Recovery from SUD is a lifelong process that often includes relapse. If the loved one and the family are progressing with the boundaries in place, there is no reason to up the ante. If there is no progress and the loved one is getting worse, the family member may need to implement more severe consequences. Rick and Jemma's daughter started drinking again, and they were able to enforce the consequence of not allowing the adult daughter to remain in their home. They did not put this boundary in place at the beginning of the recovery process because Rick, Jemma, and their coach realized that recovery included relapse. They all wanted to give group meetings, appointments, and treatment a chance to work. Just as importantly, Rick and Jemma needed time to develop the resilience, the support system, and the faith in their higher power needed to let go of their daughter and let God take care of her.

It is important to remember that Rick and Jemma enforced this boundary because they loved their daughter and they loved each other. Rick and Jemma knew that if their daughter were living with them, they would be supporting her drug use. Their daughter was paying rent, but it was minimal. The money that should have gone to rent was going to mind-altering substances. The second reason is equally essential: neither Rick nor Jemma, using their words, "… could continue to watch our daughter kill herself."

- **IT IS IMPORTANT THAT THE FAMILY MEMBER COMPLETES THEIR INVENTORY AND AMENDS STEPS—STEP 4 AND STEP 9.** For the good of the family member and the loved one, boundaries, especially the hard ones, need to be enforced from a position of kindness, love, and sadness, not anger. Completing the inventory and the amends steps allows the family member to clear away the emotional debris caused by both life and SUD in the family.

The intellectual and emotional clarity Step 4 and Step 9 bring helps the family member see their loved one as a hurting person with an awful disease. It also allows the family member to see that enforcing the boundary is kind and loving and part of the cure for the disease. As Rick often said, "Without recovery, asking my daughter to leave would have involved a lot of yelling and shaming her with statements like, 'How could you give up all we are giving you?' 'How could you do this to us?' With recovery, Rick said, 'I am sorry it has to be this way, and I love you.' His daughter said, 'I love you too, dad.'"

- **RULES AND BOUNDARIES.** There is some confusion between rules and the boundaries we discuss here. The main difference between rules and boundaries is their purpose. Rules are intended to change behavior, teach what is acceptable, and punish when broken. Boundaries are designed to protect the family, ensure the loved one feels the natural consequences of their actions, and not help the loved one use. You can also think of the boundaries we are discussing as a unique subset of rules when dealing with someone with a chemically altered mind. Unlike rules, boundaries should be enforced every time they are crossed because they deal with family safety, responding to illegal activity, and not helping a life-threatening disease progress. Boundaries can be changed through the same deliberate process used to set them.

The family member can get creative concerning the consequences if a loved one breaks a rule. A loved one refused to clean the yard, so the dad cleaned it. The loved one asked the dad for a ride to the mall, and the dad said no. The dad said he was too tired because the dad had to clean the yard. Rick and Jemma's daughter would leave her clothes all over the house. Instead of constantly yelling, Jemma started putting these clothes into the garage. Rick and Jemma's daughter finally stopped leaving her clothes around the house. One family required all their children to bring their clothes to the laundry room. Their loved one never did. The parents stopped yelling about it and stopped washing their loved one's clothes unless the clothes were in the laundry room. Eventually, the loved one had no clean clothes and started bringing his clothes to the laundry room. The key to the consequences for each of these rules is that the parents enforced them without yelling, and the consequences were the natural outcome of the loved one breaking the rule.

- **KEEP THE CONSEQUENCES CONSISTENT.** The consequences are explicitly written to make it easier for the family member and to protect the loved one. If the consequence of relapse is that the loved one needs to wait until they are 30 days sober before the family member allows the loved one to use the car, the family member should not arbitrarily raise it to 60 days. The family members can change the boundary, but they need to make the change using the boundary-setting process. It is the same for the reverse. A family member cannot arbitrarily lower the boundary. A family member reduced the number of days sober for driving because the loved one was doing so well. The son eventually relapsed. After the relapse, the son constantly badgered the father for the car, in part because the father had given in before.

- **ACCEPTING THE OUTCOME OF ENFORCING A BOUNDARY.** It is hard to describe the fear and anxiety a family member often feels when setting or enforcing a hard consequence. The fear and anxiety are about what the loved one will do or what will happen to the loved one when the family member enforces the boundary. Rick said,

> When I first started recovery, I could not set or enforce boundaries because I imagined my

daughter running away and ending up in a ditch. It was so bad that all my daughter had to do to get me to cave was say she was going for a walk. I immediately went to her being in a ditch and caved to whatever she wanted.

Getting a family member to a place where they can accept the potential outcomes requires a head and a heart-understanding of the relationship between SUD and consequences.

Having an intimate relationship with their Higher Power helps family members accept and let go of the outcome of enforcing a hard boundary. As Rick said, "Everyone was asking me to turn it over to God, but I did not have the relationship with God I needed to trust Him with my daughter." Rick worked on his relationship with God, and when the time came to enforce a hard consequence, he could let go of his daughter and let God take care of her.

- IMPOSE ONLY LEGAL AND MORAL CONSEQUENCES. This might seem self-evident, but in many cases, it is not. If your loved one owns the phone and pays for the phone service, taking the phone as a consequence is really stealing. Asking a minor to leave your home without providing them with adequate food, shelter, and clothing is illegal and unacceptable. Asking the same of an adult is both legal and acceptable.

Another example of how legality and fairness play into boundaries is what Rick and Jemma did with objectionable music. The boundary with their son was, "If we hear objectionable music, we will destroy the CD. If you bought the CD, we would replace it with a CD of your choice that does not have objectionable words. If we paid for the CD, we would not replace it." Taking and breaking a CD their son bought would be stealing, so Rick and Jemma would replace it with an unobjectionable CD. This boundary illustrates another critical point. Rick and Jemma did not give their using son cash. They went to the store with their son and paid for the CD.

> **A BOUNDARY IS NOT INTENDED TO GET THE LOVED ONE TO STOP DOING OBJECTIONABLE BEHAVIOR.** Whether to stop offensive behavior is always the loved one's choice, and this approach recognizes that fact. A boundary is not intended to get the loved one to change his behavior. As already discussed, it is designed to ensure the loved one feels the natural consequences of their behavior and to provide the family member with a well-thought-out response to objectionable behavior. This is important for some families to understand.

It is common for a family member to say boundaries do not work because the loved one is still using substances. If the family is protected, they are not enabling the loved one, and the loved one feels natural consequences, the boundaries are working.

The CD boundary Rick and Jemma had for their son also illustrates this. The boundary was based on Rick and Jemma hearing the music. They were not telling their son that he could not play the music. Rick and Jemma did not want to listen to the music. This was about their sanity and not about trying to control what their son was listening to. Would Rick and Jemma have preferred their son not to listen to this degrading music? Of course! Rick and Jemma knew that getting their son to stop listening was an effort to control their son.

- **IF THE LOVED ONE IS IN RECOVERY, THE LOVED ONE KNOWS ENFORCING A BOUNDARY IS THE RIGHT THING TO DO.** Even as the loved one is loudly objecting, they know that enforcing a boundary is what needs to happen. In general, as enforcing boundaries becomes the norm, the loved one's anger begins to be replaced by acceptance and, perhaps, respect for the family member. Butch had to enforce a hard boundary on his adult son. The adult son, James, relapsed, and the consequence was that the adult son had to move out of the house. James' sisters called Butch and complained about Butch asking his son to move out. Butch found out later that James called each of his siblings and told them that Butch was doing the right thing. James did not like what was happening, but he knew Butch was doing the right thing and was doing it from a position of kindness and love.

CHAPTER 11

Resent, Own, Appreciate, Demand (ROAD) Tool

The Resent, Own, Appreciate, Demand (ROAD) tool is an inventory tool PDAP and other organizations use to address resentments. ROAD can be used as a part of the AA 4th Step inventory process, or it can be used independently to address resentments as they arise. In this book, ROAD is used to help family members work through resentments that are blocking the family member's recovery. A modification of the ROAD can be used to lovingly confront a person crossing a family member's boundary. The objectives of this chapter are to:

- Outline the ROAD process and illustrate its use.
- Show how family members can use ROAD to deal with lingering resentments.
- Show how family members can use ROAD to confront someone lovingly.

Appendix J: Resent, Own, Appreciate, Demand (ROAD) Worksheet can be given to a family member as an exercise to work through the ROAD process. The worksheet will not be discussed question by question because the discussion below mirrors the worksheet.

The ROAD Process

The primary application of ROAD is dealing with past resentments that are still blocking a family member's recovery. We will use George's story about his dad, John, to illustrate the ROAD process.

John, George's father, was a good man suffering from the disease of alcoholism. Like most adult children of alcoholics, George carried resentments about his father's drinking into adulthood. George and his wife Anne had five wonderful children, and their lives together were wonderful until, in 1995, two of George and Anne's children started using substances and rapidly progressed to severe SUD. In 1996, George, Anne, and their two loved ones entered PDAP and started their respective recovery journeys. George worked the 12 Steps three times from start to finish. George's recovery from codependence was of the "sometimes slowly" variety. However, George believed his resentments were well controlled after the third inventory.

In 1999, John wanted to visit George, Anne, and, more importantly, his grandchildren. George made it clear that his house was now a non-drinking house and asked his dad not to drink while he visited. George's two loved ones were in the initial stages of their recovery, and the smell of alcohol was a trigger for both of George's loved ones.

The visit went well. John did not drink, or if he did, George did not notice. It was time for John to fly home. George and Anne took John to the airport, wished him well, and then headed home happy about how well the visit went. Shortly after George and Anne arrived home, John called to say his flight was canceled. George drove back to the airport, and as soon as John got in the car, George smelled alcohol and was silently furious. George recounted this incident for several years as an example of John crossing a boundary. For all these years, George remained silently, self-righteously furious. This changed when George attended a ROAD workshop.

RESENT

In the first step of the ROAD process, ask the family member to name the person who hurt them and what that person did with specificity. It is helpful to ask the family members to close their eyes, imagine the person who hurt them, and then review what actually occurred. Then, like the AA 4th Step inventory process, the family member will write the person's name, what the person did to the family member, and how it made the family member feel. The family member must describe what the person did with specificity.

At the ROAD workshop, George was asked to identify a specific resentment. George's first response was, "I resent my dad's drinking, and it made me feel angry." While this was true, it was not specific enough. George thought for a bit and wrote, "I resent my dad for drinking during his visit to our house after I specifically asked my dad not to. It made me feel angry." This was specific, but the coach asked for more specificity. Frustrated, George wrote, "I resent my dad for drinking at the airport while he was waiting for his flight home. It made me feel furious, manipulated, and betrayed." When George read what he wrote to his coach, something clicked. He realized his dad respected George's boundaries. John did not drink while at George's house. John drank at the airport when he believed he was on his way home. John had no way of knowing that the airline would cancel his flight. Unfortunately, George could not make amends because John died before the workshop. George's story illustrates the importance of discussing the resentment with the family member to ensure the family member is aware of the actual cause. In George's case, George was the cause of George's resentment. George had a faulty belief about what his dad did. His dad did respect George's boundaries.

OWN

The "O" or own in ROAD asks the family members to examine the event and own their part. What was the family member's part in the interaction that hurt him? As illustrated by George's story above, at times, a faulty belief was the family member's part in the resentment. Other examples of actions a family member can own include:

- **JUMPING TO CONCLUSIONS.** George jumped to the conclusion that his dad violated his boundary because George smelled alcohol on his dad's breath. George could have asked clarifying questions or could have thought the situation through.

- **HOLDING ON TO RESENTMENTS.** George had a lingering resentment against his father's drinking. The smell of alcohol triggered the unresolved resentment that took George straight to, as it turned out, unjustified anger. A coach discussing the "O" in ROAD talked about the resentment against her father for abusing her when she was young. The coach had no part in the abuse because she was a child. What she owned was that she used the resentment as an excuse to continue her substance use.

- **TRUSTING A LOVED ONE BEFORE HE IS TRUSTWORTHY.** A family group member shared the following, "I allowed my daughter to stay at a friend's house when she was in early recovery. She came home high, and I was angry. Yes, I was angry at her for being high, but I was also angry at myself for trusting her when I knew she was not trustworthy."

- **SAYING "YES" WHEN YOU MEAN "NO."** A family group member relayed the following story. "I was sitting at the table with my daughter, and she asked me to take her to see a friend. I blew up. I got angry and started scolding her. When I took a breath, she said, 'You could have said no.' I was speechless because she was right. My daughter asked for a ride, but I was the one who said yes. I should have been mad at myself and not my daughter." It is essential that family members understand that it is okay to say "no" to something just because the family member does not want to do it. The family group member's resentment grew each time she said yes to her daughter when she really wanted to say no.

- **FAILING TO ENFORCE A BOUNDARY.** Failing to enforce a boundary can lead to guilt if things go wrong. For example, a parent/guardian lets a loved one drive a car after being ten days sober when the boundary was that the loved one needed to be 30 days sober. If the loved one gets into an accident and is high, the parent/guardian bears some responsibility for the event. If nothing else, the parent/guardian's guilt over not enforcing the boundary will exacerbate their reaction to the accident.

- **OTHER EXAMPLES OF OWN INCLUDE:**
  - "I own that I got angry and said some hurtful things that I should not have said when I found out you lied."
  - "I own that I did not call my sponsor before confronting you."
  - "I own that I used what you did as an excuse to stay in my codependence."
  - "I own that my self-centeredness was a part of this."

APPRECIATE

The appreciate step is where the family member can express gratitude for any lesson learned, express understanding if there are any mitigating circumstances, and express understanding if they did something similar in the past. Each of these will ease the charge associated with the resentment. Examples of "appreciate" statements:

- "I was a teenager once and appreciate how you would want to go to a party with your girlfriend."
- "I appreciate that your relapse was, in part, a response to your girlfriend breaking up with you."
- "I appreciate that you were very tired when you started yelling at me."
- "I appreciate the lesson I learned about not enforcing a boundary. As you demonstrated when you lied to me, the boundaries are in place for a good reason."
- "I appreciate the validation of my judgment. I knew you were not yet trustworthy, and I was correct."
- "I appreciate that I lied to my parents as a teenager. Like now, there were consequences for my lying."
- "I appreciate the character defects that were identified in me. I was selfish because I wanted to be the good parent."
- "I appreciate that I did this to someone else."
- "I appreciate that I have lied to you in the past."

The appreciate step does not absolve the loved one of their wrongdoing. The appreciate step makes forgiving easier because of the mitigating circumstances or because the family member has done similar things in the past and wanted forgiveness.

DEMAND

The demand statement is made for each resentment: "I demand that you stop." When dealing with resentments, the demand step clarifies that the past cannot be changed. If the hurtful behavior is ongoing, the demand statement can be turned into a boundary using the methodology in Chapter 10, Boundaries for Families Dealing with Substance Use Disorder.

ROAD USED TO LOVINGLY CONFRONT

ROAD is also a tool to confront someone hurting the family member in the present. In this case, the ROAD is used to get the person to stop hurting the family member or crossing a family member's boundary. The ROAD approach defuses the situation, fosters understanding, and facilitates change in the offender. As shown in Appendix J: Resent, Own, Appreciate, Demand (ROAD) Worksheet, the process for using ROAD in a confrontation is the same except for the last step. The final step is enforcing the boundary if a boundary is in place or, if there is no boundary, setting a boundary.

Parting Thoughts on ROAD

ROAD is a tool for helping rid family members of their resentments toward the people who hurt them. It is one of many that can help family members with one of the most essential parts of recovery—forgiving the people who hurt them.

The family member must understand that forgiving someone does not mean they trust them, like them, or want to be in a relationship with them. It does mean that the person no longer has the power to ruin the family member's day just by being in the same room. It means the family member no longer cringes when they see them or cringe when they think of them. It means the person is no longer "living rent-free in the family member's head."

The ROAD process aids in forgiving past hurts because the "own" and "appreciate" helps the family member gain compassion for their loved one. The "own" can help the family member identify their part in the event. Taking ownership of their contribution helps to take some of the sting out of the event. Often, what the family member "owns" is their misunderstanding of the disease of SUD. Working to provide the family member with a head-heart-understanding of the disease helps here.

The "appreciate" can help the family member to see the whole picture more clearly. Appreciating that the relapse occurred after a traumatic event or after an extended period of sobriety helps to reframe the event. "Appreciate" can also help the family members recognize that they have done similar things.

The purpose of the own and appreciate steps is to help bring compassion into the family member's heart and voice. It is not to absolve the person of what they did wrong. It is not a means to justify mitigating the consequences of your loved one's actions. Sometimes, a family member will say, "I use drugs, so how can I enforce boundaries when my loved one uses drugs." This false argument falls under the line "Two wrongs do not make a right." Disclose your past similar actions only if the disclosure helps accomplish the objective of confrontation.

CHAPTER 12

Living in the Moment

Worrying about the future and regretting the past can rob the moment's serenity. Living in the moment is a skill that builds resilience and allows the family members to have periods where they can enjoy life. Like many recovery tools, learning and applying living in the moment is a three-step process. First is understanding the concept or a "head-understanding." The second is a "heart-understanding," where the family member believes in the tool. The third is using the tool and learning how to use it well. The objectives of this chapter are to provide:

- An understanding of living in the moment and its benefits.
- A methodology to facilitate a family member walking through the three steps—head-understanding, heart-understanding, and using the tool.

What is Living in the Moment?

The living in-the-moment tool helps a family member focus on what their life is like in the present moment. It means not living in the past by constantly rehashing past events. "If I had done it this way, things would have been much better." "I wish I said this when he said that." These are all examples of living in the past. Two of the most detrimental forms of past-living are holding on to and nurturing resentments and holding on to and nurturing shame. Living in the future is living as if the events the family member fears will happen, have already occurred. A mom feeling the sadness of a loved one's death even though he is still alive. A dad worrying about the impact of a loved one's arrest on the loved one's future, even though the loved one has not yet been arrested. A mom is anxious and upset during her drive home from work because she fears what awaits her: a loved one acting out, a message from the school, or even the police at the door.

Living in the moment is completely experiencing the immediate present and doing the next right thing the immediate present calls for. The mom's car ride home is a scenario that illustrates living in the moment. Most family members have lived through this scenario. While the mom was on her drive, none of the things she was worried about were occurring. She was feeling fear and anxiety because the mom chose to think about what could be waiting for her when she got home. If the mom *decided* to think about the scenery, chose to think about the song on the radio, or decided to do a gratitude list, she would not be feeling the fear her negative thoughts were generating. Instead of arriving home tense, fearful, and exhausted, the mom could arrive home relaxed, refreshed, and ready to respond to whatever was happening at home.

Sometimes, the past and the future require actions "in the now." For example, if the past still haunts you, it is time "in the now" to do an inventory to forgive those who hurt you and make amends to those you hurt. Another example is planning. Planning for the future is an action needed "in the now." Planning for the future differs from worrying about the future or living as if a future disaster has already occurred. Having a recovery plan and setting boundaries are things a family member needs to do in the "now" to plan for the future.

Using Appendix K: Living in the Moment

The living in the moment worksheet (Appendix K: Living in the Moment) gives the family member a methodology to live in the moment. The following discussion provides guidance for each question in the worksheet.

QUESTION 1 asks the family member to do a feelings check and write down their feelings in the moment. QUESTION 2 asks the family member to identify what was generating the feelings. The purpose of the feelings check is to start having the family member identify past and future issues that infringe on the family member's ability to live in the moment fully. Take note of the reasons for the feelings. Are the reasons in the past, present, or the future? The simple statement, "I am nervous," is not helpful unless the family member explains the reason for being nervous. "I am nervous because I am thinking about when I failed to get the promotion I deserved." This is a past issue. I am nervous because this is the first appointment with you." This is an in-the-moment issue. "I am nervous because the loved one is home alone." This is a future issue because the family member is nervous about what might happen. Listening to the whys for the feelings and then parsing them into the past, the moment, and the future helps explain the concept.

QUESTION 3 asks the family member to read the poem " Where *Are You?* by Eric Daxon and then write down what the poem says to them.[18] The poem tries to tie several points together. First, you can only control what you do in the "now." In the now, the person in the poem needed to let go of the past, not dwell on the future and rest. Second, the circumstances might be dire, but there are moments that the family members can and should enjoy. The poem implies

---

[18] We wanted to include the poem *I Am* by Helen Mallicoat in the appendix, but we could not determine who held the copyright for the poem. (Mallicoat 2020) Eric Daxon wrote *Where Are You?* as a poor substitute for *I Am* to try to get Ms. Mallicoat's point across.

that the person in the poem, Joseph, was having financial problems. However, it was night, he was not hungry in the moment, and he was not homeless in the moment. If he had already planned for the next day, he had nothing more to do. At that moment, he was not hungry, had shelter, and knew what he would do. In the moment, nothing was wrong except his choice to worry. Third, God can and will remove the anxiety if asked to and if the person believes God can.

QUESTION 4 asks the family member to examine the current moment carefully and determine if anything is amiss. Ask them to describe the exact moment they are in, where they are sitting, what they are doing, who is in the room with them, and whether it is comfortable. If they are worried about their loved one, ask them if their loved one is in the room. When they are in an appointment, there is nothing in the present that could take away their serenity. If they have financial issues, ask them if they are hungry, lack shelter, or lack clothing right now.

Sitting in your office, the answer should be "no." Several things will make the answer "yes." All will be about the distant and immediate past or the immediate and distant future. One of the roadblocks to enjoying the moment is the false belief that it is inappropriate for family members to enjoy themselves when their loved one has SUD. This belief is counter to the fun component of our culture. It can be helpful to frame the necessity of the family member enjoying the moments of peace as enabling the loved one's recovery and enabling the family member's recovery. Enjoying those moments of serenity refreshes and builds the resilience the family member will need to face the next crisis. This enables a loved one's recovery because a resilient, refreshed family member is more likely to enforce boundaries, let go, and be kind to their loved one.

QUESTION 5 is based on Dawn's story, which is as follows:

> After one of our most challenging seasons with our teens, I frequently thought about how horrible the whole year was, and it kept me feeling so heavy and so sad. But when I challenged myself to consider how many terrible days there were ... days with fighting [with her teen] or [her teen] sneaking out or

getting a call from the school...there were thirty? Sixty? And that left three hundred medium and even good days to focus on. That shift in perspective eventually helped me view our life and our child in a more positive light, even as our struggles continued.

Sometimes, all it takes for a family member to enjoy the moment is the ability to recognize the serenity in the moment. Dawn's story highlights that there were many moments of relative calm and even happiness in one of the worst periods of her teen's SUD. Dawn did not notice them and did not fully enjoy them. Dawn's story and the following questions attempt to open the family members to the possibility that they can enjoy moments during a crisis because they have already enjoyed them. They did not notice these joy-filled moments. The sub-bullets to the question ask the family members to write their version of Dawn's story.

The first sub-bullet asks the family members to remember and write down the story they tell others about their life since SUD entered the family. Usually, this story recounts the trauma and crisis SUD brought to the family. The second sub-bullet asks the family members to write down how their story makes them feel. Dawn felt heavy and sad.

The third sub-bullet asks if there were any good times since SUD entered the family. Remembering the good times may require prompting. Laughing during a meeting or outing indicates that family members are having fun. For an enthusiastic golfer, golfing is likely an enjoyable time. The family member does not necessarily forget these fun times, but the fun times are hidden in a different box when the family member discusses SUD in the family. The recovery coach's job is to open the box and help integrate the contents into the totality of the family member's memory. Recognizing that one has been happy in the middle of a crisis before makes it easier to use and trust the Living in the Moment tool.

QUESTION 6 asks the family member to act as if they were able, in the moment, to let go of regretting the past and let go of worrying about the future.

This is also a suitable time for the recovery coach to share their experience with living in the moment. The tendency at this point is to dump or say they feel fine. If someone says they are feeling fine, ask them to think about a moment in the past when they were worrying, anxious, or depressed. The key is to get them to acknowledge that regretting the past and worrying about the future generates feelings that rob them of the moment's serenity. The last part of the question asks the family members to reflect on the good times they identified in QUESTION 5.

Parting Thoughts on Living in the Moment

Living in the past and living in the future are also coping mechanisms because the family member does not yet have the tools and support needed to live solidly in the present. This coping mechanism does have benefits:

- Not having to deal with what was going on in the present. For example, worrying about what could happen gives an acceptable excuse to slack off at work.

- Feeling like a martyr such that people will either feel sorry for them or praise them. Sympathy and praise are powerful motivators for a family member who is depressed and full of anxiety.

- Regretting the past often feels like atonement for what happened in the past without ever having to make amends.

- Anxiety and depression were proof of their love for their loved ones.

It is essential that the family members experience what living in the moment feels like even before they are ready to do so. The first time most family members experience or witness the gift of living in the moment is in a meeting. Their loved one is not with them, and in many cases, their loved one is in their own meeting and safe. Coffee afterward also forces the person to live in the moment. The "old-timers" are typically good at helping people enjoy coffee. Activities are another place to experience living in the moment, especially if the family member's loved one is also at a separate activity.

CHAPTER 13

Strengthening a Relationship with God

One of the purposes of the 12 Steps of AA or any other 12-Step program is to build an understanding of and a relationship with a Higher Power. An ever-deepening belief in a Higher Power is the glue that holds the Steps together and the force that empowers family members to do the challenging work the 12 Steps ask us to do. Everyone comes to their first meeting or appointment with their own relationship with a Higher Power. These relationships range from a strong belief in the Abrahamic God to the atheistic belief that a God or Higher Power does not exist.

The objectives of this chapter are to:

- Provide tools to overcome the fear that often infuses every aspect of a family member's life, whether they believe in a Higher Power or not.

- Provide tools that allow those with a belief in a Higher Power to deepen their relationship with that Higher Power.

- Provide those who do not believe in a Higher Power the ability to explore the possibility that a Higher Power does exist and come to a new understanding of who or what their Higher Power might be.

Gratitude Lists

Writing a gratitude list is the simplest and sometimes the most effective tool for bringing relief, whether the family member has a Higher Power or not. In the middle of the tough times that accompany SUD, it is easy for a family member to focus on what is going wrong to the extent that they forget what is good in their lives. Gratitude lists help family members remember the good things in their lives. In addition to recognizing the good, gratitude lists provide a respite from the misery the family member may feel. Misery and gratitude cannot coexist. This process provides relief, not usually long-term relief, but relief. This may be the first time the family member feels relief since SUD entered their home. Gratitude lists also foster a close and intimate relationship with their Higher Power.

There are multiple ways to do gratitude lists. One effective way is to ask the client to write down ten things they are grateful for each day using the following guidelines:

- DO NOT SHOW THE LIST TO ANYONE. This is between the family member and their Higher Power. This fosters both honesty and intimacy with their Higher Power. For most, knowing someone else would read the list will change what and how they write the gratitude list. Eric's story illustrates this:

    When my sponsor told me to do a daily gratitude list, I thought it was odd that he admonished me not to show it to anyone, not even my sponsor. The last part puzzled me even more. Not showing it to my sponsor seemed to go against what the sponsor/sponsee relationship was supposed to be. I thought about it for a while, and then it hit me. If I knew I would show someone my gratitude list, I would make it the best one they ever saw! (Can you tell that false pride was one of my character defects?)

Keeping it between God and me fostered honesty with myself and God. Some days when I was particularly down, my gratitude list was basic—grateful I could see, hear, etc. Admitting this period of ungratefulness to myself and God created a feeling of intimacy with God that I had not felt in a long time.

- **IT MUST BE TEN THINGS.** Requiring ten helps when times are hard, and there is not much to be grateful for. Sometimes, the gratitude list is lovely, and sometimes, it is basic ("I have eyes; I have food; I can walk; I can hear.") Even a basic gratitude list can bring relief.

- **WRITE THE LIST IN A JOURNAL.** Being able to reread gratitude lists helps in a couple of ways. First, it can give a lift when people are down. Second, it shows that they can have relief anytime they want relief. Third, writing the list allows the family members to think about what they are writing, write what they are thinking, and then read what they wrote. This process engages multiple senses and helps internalize the gratitude the family member expresses.

Unlike the daily gratitude list, one can start a spontaneous gratitude list anytime. It does not need to be written, nor does it need to be ten items. One purpose of spontaneous gratitude lists is for the family member to enter a conversation with God. This is a way for the family member to "...improve their conscious contact..." with God. The second purpose of a spontaneous gratitude list is to help a family member get out of a codependent relapse.

One of the most difficult codependent relapses to recover from is being on a "pity pot." In recovery circles, a pity pot is when someone revels in all that is going wrong in their life. A person often will relish thinking about how life has been so unfair. A spontaneous gratitude list can break this cycle. Remembering the good things and enjoying the feelings associated with the good things in their lives will displace the misery of a pity pot. It helps if the family member understands that this can be a quick or slow process, but it will work if the family member continues the gratitude list until the misery is gone. In more colloquial terms, continue the gratitude list until you want to, and do, get off the pity pot.

Using Appendix L: AA Big Book Prayers, Your Higher Power Speaking to You

The AA Big Book Prayers, Your Higher Power Speaking to You, on page 341, uses the AA Third Step Prayer and Seventh Step Prayer to explore and deepen the family member's relationship with his Higher Power. The worksheet is for family members already seeking a deeper relationship with their Higher Power or family members you believe would be open to this. Ideally, they are working on the steps with a sponsor. The worksheet may be counterproductive for clients who consider themselves atheists or agnostics. Please be aware that the worksheet's questions may trigger past trauma.

The worksheet has three sections. The first two sections, Third Step Prayer and Seventh Step Prayer have questions for the family members about these specific prayers. The last section, Questions Related to Both Prayers, not surprisingly has questions related to both prayers.

AA BIG BOOK THIRD STEP PRAYER

The worksheet questions for the Third Step Prayer are to aid the family member in identifying the character defects that are blocking them from making a real decision to turn their will and lives over to God's care as they understand him. (Alcoholics Anonymous 2019) Often, family members will confuse the decision to submit to God with actually turning their will and their lives over to God. If this is the case, it is important to highlight that the third step is deciding to and not actually accomplishing it.

A story to illustrate the difference is building a building. A contractor decides to construct a building. Is the building built? No. Once the contractor decides to build, they must work to make it a reality. The work includes buying the land, getting the permits, hiring an architect, buying the materials, hiring the laborers, overcoming problems encountered, and getting the building inspected. The decision is just the start of the process of turning our will and lives over to God's care as we understand Him.

QUESTION 1 asks specifically about the message they received the first time they read the prayer and the message God is sending in the present. It is essential to guide the family member away from talking about how they felt and toward discussing what their Higher Power told them after they read the prayer for the first time and what their Higher Power is telling them now. The purpose behind this is to reinforce that God does communicate with us and to determine how to differentiate their thoughts from God communicating with them.

QUESTION 2 asks the family member what "shackles" prevent them from acting on their decision in Step 3. The first answer many give is time—they must devote more time to prayer and meditation. Lack of time is a pat answer that rarely is the actual shackle. Here are some common shackles:

- **THEY DO NOT TRUST GOD.** As one anonymous parent with a loved one in active addiction put it, "They asked me to trust God. Why would I trust God? From where I am sitting, He has messed it up so far!" The usually unspoken part of this statement is that the family members do not trust God to do what they want God to do. This reveals the second typical shackle:

- **PRIDE AND ARROGANCE.** Not trusting God because God did not do what the family member wanted God to do means the family member knew what was best and God did not. A family member knowing better is quite common in Stage 1 and Stage 2 codependency, where the family member's self-will is still intact. Remember, this is pride and arrogance, either born or stoked by fear.

- **OVERWHELMING FEAR.** Fear drives people to act or prevents them from acting. Turning your will and your life over to the care of God means accepting that the next right thing to do may be to do nothing. It takes tremendous courage for a family member to do nothing when fear for their loved one is all-consuming. It also takes immense courage for a family member to overcome paralyzing fear and do the next right thing.

- **A LACK OF UNDERSTANDING.** It is hard to turn your will and life over to the care of someone you do not understand. This is more than not understanding who God is; it is not understanding what a Higher Power means. This understanding needs to be both taught and experienced.

AA BIG BOOK SEVENTH STEP PRAYER

The Seventh Step Prayer includes two essential concepts for recovery in general and especially for family members. (Alcoholics Anonymous 2019) Specifically:

- **GOD REMOVES THE CHARACTER DEFECTS.** It is common to hear a family member say, "I am doing all of this work, and it is not working." It is essential that they understand that their job is to do their recovery work, and it is up to God to remove the defect. There is usually great relief when the family member finally understands God decides when to remove the defect. One family member said, "I am relieved. I thought I was doing it wrong. I need to keep working and wait for God."

- **CHARACTER DEFECTS ARE REMOVED TO ENHANCE SERVICE.** Removing character defects improves the client's usefulness to God but does not necessarily make the client happy. When dealing with a codependent family member, it is important to stress the need for self-care and the need to let others solve their own problems.

QUESTIONS 1 and 2 get the client thinking about the prayer, the messages they received when they first read it, and the message now. QUESTION 3 is important because it addresses acceptance. Many will answer "No" because they believe acceptance means being satisfied with who they are. A "no" answer provides an opportunity to talk about the real meaning of acceptance, which is recognizing who the family member is in the moment and accepting that as reality. The key sub-question in QUESTION 3 is, "Do you have a choice?" The off-the-cuff answer is "No." The honest answer is "Yes." The client can ignore their defects or refuse to do the work that will elucidate these hidden/unnoticed character defects. QUESTION 3 also brings out several other key points:

- **ACCEPTANCE OF SELF.** Self-acceptance is a crucial aspect of recovery culture. Becoming willing to give God the person that the family member is in the moment requires them to accept—not necessarily approve of—the person they are in the moment.

- **CLARITY ABOUT SELF.** The prayer acknowledges that each of us has strengths and weaknesses and calls us to eschew false pride—thinking we are better than we are. It also calls on us to shun false humility—thinking we are worse than we are.

- **THEY DESERVE GOD'S LOVE.** Giving the bad to our Higher Power is a tacit admission that we know that our Higher Power loves us and accepts us. The real "us."

- **GOD'S WILL IS IMPORTANT AND NOT MY WILL.** The last part of the prayer requires the admission that God's will for us is essential. The strength asked for in the prayer is to seek God's will and subjugate self-will to God's will.

QUESTIONS RELATED TO BOTH THE AA THIRD STEP AND SEVENTH STEP PRAYERS

QUESTION 1 asks the family member to look for the common themes in both prayers. The first sub-bullet asks the family members to identify the common themes in each prayer. If the family member is stuck, the following are some of the major themes running through both prayers:

- **MAKING A CONSCIOUS CHOICE TO SUBMIT TO GOD.** The first sentence in the Third Step Prayer is about offering ourselves to God. The Seventh Step Prayer repeats the offering and indicates a willingness to do so. It is common to decide and not be willing to carry it out. The sequence is important—decide, become willing, and, as we will see in Step 11, take steps to carry through on the decision made.

- **ADMITTING POWERLESSNESS.** Both prayers include an admission of being powerless over what they cannot control. The Third Step Prayer recognizes our inability to free ourselves from the "bondage of self." It also recognizes our inability to remove problems because we do not control outcomes. The Seventh Step Prayer reinforces that by asking God to remove our character defects. We are powerless to change ourselves.

- **WE MUST DO OUR PART.** We control what we say, what we do, what we believe, what we think, and what we feel. In the Third Step Prayer, our action is, with sincerity, turning ourselves over to God and choosing to serve others—"... bear witness *to those I would help*..." We choose to believe that God is trustworthy and will, in His time and in His way, relieve us of the bondage of self and our hardships. The Seventh Step Prayer requires us to become willing to believe that, as it says in the AA Big Book on page 84, "God can and will do for us what we could not do for ourselves" (Alcoholics Anonymous 2019). The last action this prayer asks for is doing God's will.

- **GOD IS ESSENTIAL IN OVERCOMING ADVERSITY.** The Third Step Prayer asks God to take away our difficulties. The Seventh Step Prayer asks God to remove character defects and provide the strength to do God's will.

- **CHOOSING TO LET GO OF SELF-WILL AND DO GOD'S WILL.** The Third Step Prayer asks God to remove self-will and self-interest by removing "...the bondage of self." The Seventh Step Prayer asks for strength to do God's bidding. The Eleventh Step discussion in the next section discusses supplanting our will with God's will.

- **CHOOSING TO BE OF SERVICE TO OTHERS.** This is a foreshadowing of AA Step 12: "Having had a spiritual awakening as a result of these Steps, we tried to carry this message to other alcoholics and to practice these principles in all our affairs."

The second sub-bullet asks the family members to consider their success in implementing these themes. The responses range from being too hard on themselves ("I have not implemented any") to being very defensive ("Yes, I did them all" or "I missed some because..."). This question aims to uncover the roadblocks (next sub-bullet) to adopting the faith and trust in God required to do the actions in each of these prayers. The last sub-bullet asks the family members to imagine their lives if they could overcome these roadblocks and trust God.

QUESTION 2 asks about new insights about themselves, their relationship with God, and God's love for them. The two prayers outlined the completeness of submission to God and His will. This is the time for a family member to have a real gut check about the intimacy of their relationship with God, a gut check on how much they trust their Higher Power, and a gut check of how much power the family member believes their Higher Power has.

The last gut check is crucial because it drives a family member's ability to let go of their loved one. Eric had trouble letting go because of how powerless his Higher Power was. Eric was science-trained and, to a certain extent, bought into the argument that reason and logic were sufficient. Eric described his initial understanding of God as,

> God was like a good friend. Sometimes, I needed his help. Sometimes, He needed mine. I was okay trusting a friend if things were going well. My trust in God all but evaporated when my family and my marriage were threatened. In times like these, I trusted myself. My family and my marriage were too important to turn it over to a friend.

Eric had to be humbled by his bottom before he came to believe in God as a real Higher Power.

QUESTION 3 focuses the family members on God's love for them. It is hard to trust someone you believe does not love you. The worksheet tries to get the family members to focus on God's love for them using the anonymous quote, "You will never look into the eyes of someone God does not love." Generally, a family member will read the quote and think of their loved one. Asking the family members to look at their own eyes in a mirror redirects them to think about God loving them. Ask the family members to dwell on God loving, really loving them. The family member choosing to believe God loves them is critical for strengthening the family member's relationship with their Higher Power.

Using Appendix M: Prayer and Meditation

Prayer and meditation are some of the most essential tools for a family member. Sometimes, a family member can pray but cannot or does not want to meditate. The same is true for prayer. Used alone, each provides important benefits. The benefit is more than doubled if used together. First, both provide a way to detach from the chaos in the home. This allows experiencing the benefits of detaching, making it easier to detach from the more complicated things—their loved one, spouse, or partner.

Second, both allow the unconscious brain to work on the problem because they will enable the family member to detach from the day's worries. The relationship between a family member and their Higher Power is the most critical determinant of the family member's ability to let go of their loved one and become willing to let go of their character defects.

The worksheet in Appendix M: Prayer and Meditation guides the family member through a series of questions that will make the family member aware of their current prayer and meditation practices and encourage improvement. The worksheet asks the family member to examine their current prayer and meditation practices in "Examine Your Prayer" and "Examine Your Meditation." This worksheet assumes that the family member has completed Appendix L: AA Big Book Prayers, Your Higher Power Speaking to You.

This worksheet is for clients already seeking a deeper relationship or clients you believe would be open to this. This worksheet may be counterproductive for clients who consider themselves atheists or agnostics because of the emphasis on prayer and God. One workaround is to modify the worksheet to address meditation. Be aware of the potential for these questions to trigger past trauma.

This worksheet has three sections. The first section, Prayer and Meditation, has questions concerning the family member's prayer and meditation. The following two sections, Examine Your Prayer and Examine Your Meditation, have questions designed to facilitate a deeper understanding of prayer and meditation as tools for building a more intimate relationship with their Higher Power.

PRAYER AND MEDITATION

QUESTION 1 asks the family member to describe how their experience with prayer and meditation has changed since the start of their recovery. This question serves two purposes. First, it starts the family member thinking about their prayer and meditation in a neutral manner. Second, it guides the family members to specifically examine how their prayer meditation practices have changed and, hopefully, become more meaningful. Sometimes, family members lose sight of their progress, especially when the family is in crisis. Reminding them of their progress offers hope. If the family member is in early recovery (less than 3 months), the question asks them to describe their current prayer and meditation and then describe what they would like their prayer and meditation to be.

QUESTION 2 addresses the family member's roadblocks that hinder prayer and meditation. For those early in recovery, it might be just ignorance. A common roadblock a family member will name is time. This usually is not the real roadblock. The real roadblock is causing them to discount meditation to the point that they are unwilling to incorporate it into their day. Some more common roadblocks include believing prayer and meditation do not work or thinking there is no value to prayer and meditation. Please take note of the real roadblocks and address them as you continue reviewing the worksheet.

QUESTION 3 and QUESTION 4 are two sides of the same coin. QUESTION 3 asks what the family member gains by not praying and meditating daily. QUESTION 4 asks what they will gain by praying and meditating daily. The easy answer to QUESTION 3 is that they will gain time. Many will also gain by being true to their beliefs. Many believe that prayer and meditation do not work and are only for religious people. One "gain" from not praying and meditating, not often mentioned, is that the family members can remain in the misery they believe they deserve. If the family member struggles with QUESTION 4, the recovery coach can share their experience. This is an excellent point to stress that the benefits of prayer and meditation come "...sometimes quickly, sometimes slowly."

Eric Daxon tells a story that illustrates this. Mr. Smith (fictitious name for a real person) was the father of Eric's close friend. Mr. Smith was trying to convert Eric to be a Lutheran, and for his final argument, Mr. Smith said, "Eric, when I have a difficult phone call to make. I pray for God to give me the words. Then I pick up the phone, dial the number, and the words are there." Eric's internal response was, "This guy is crazy. That is not how it works. I need to get away from this guy!" As Eric relays the story, "I always remembered that interaction and the certainty I felt that prayer was useless. I carried that skepticism into recovery and held on to it for a long time until I hit my bottom. I asked God for relief from the agony, and relief came. Now, I am Mr. Smith. I do pray for the words before tough conversations. Prayer and meditation are now an integral part of my daily life."

QUESTION 5 asks what the family member thinks St. Francis de Sales meant when he said, "Every one of us needs half an hour of prayer a day, except when we are busy—then we need an hour." This quote gets to the second reason: prayer and meditation are essential. In addition to improving our relationship with our Higher Power, prayer and meditation are time enhancers rather than time wasters. Prayer and meditation restore the emotional reserves needed to effectively live a life severely impacted by SUD in the home. The peace and calm from prayer and meditation provide the ability to see the most critical tasks for the day.

QUESTION 6 asks what the family member thinks St. Teresa of Calcutta meant when she said, "I used to believe that prayer changes things, but now I know that prayer changes us, and we change things." This is a direct analog to the last half of Step 11—"...praying only for knowledge of His will for us and the power to carry that out."[19]

This statement reinforces the need for family members to be in recovery because it clarifies that the family member needs to take an active part in changing themselves first. Then, they will have the ability to change their circumstances.

EXAMINE YOUR PRAYER

QUESTION 1 gets to the critical aspect by asking the family member to write down the most intimate thing the family member has shared with God. The most common statement by a family member is, "God knows everything. Why do I need to tell Him?" The family member's Higher Power may know everything, but intimacy is based on two-way, honest communication. Their Higher Power does not need to hear it, but they need to share it. It is important to ask the family member about the emotions and feelings he experienced while answering this question. The level of intimacy in the sharing and the strength of the feelings felt while answering the question help to set a baseline for the family member's relationship with God.

---

19 Some 12 Step traditions use "courage" in place of "power" so the last half of Step 11 would read, "...praying only for knowledge of His will for us and the *courage* to carry that out."

QUESTION 2 takes QUESTION 1 deeper by explicitly asking about areas the client is "hiding" from their Higher Power. The first sub-question is about being dishonest with God. The most usual form of dishonesty is not expressing anger toward God. The second most common is the pledge to change without taking the action to change. Rote prayers are good unless the family member uses them to tick a box. In this instance, they are blocking intimacy. Walled-off areas are usually shame-based. The best example is pornography for men. Walling off can also be the result of trauma.

QUESTION 3 asks the family member to identify the feelings they have hidden from God. One measure of intimacy in a relationship is sharing the full range of feelings with the person. This question aims to foster a more open sharing of feelings with God as soon as they occur. The approach is a modification of the approach used for the Step 4 inventory. One of the examples in QUESTION 3 will be used to explain the "hidden-feelings inventory."

The sub-question asks the family member to name the feelings they are hiding from God. A familiar feeling is anger at God. Second, it asks the family member to select the most important feeling and write about it as if they were sharing the feeling with God. The worksheet provides an example from a family group member's recovery story. Usually, the feeling is associated with an event or action that the family member knows was wrong. In the example listed in QUESTION 3, the event was the family member becoming inebriated when the intent was to have just one drink. The example shows how sharing the hidden feeling (compulsion to drink) led to what was at the root of not wanting to share with God (shame and guilt), which was followed by further isolation from God ("I was convinced I could control it the next time."). The next part is how the family member wants to respond in the future when the desire to hide from God comes again (share the feeling with God and another person).

Usually, there is more behind this that the family member has not shared with God. In the family member's case, not sharing the compulsion to drink led to the realization that there were other feelings/events that he/she was not sharing with God. The insecurity he/she felt at work. The anxiety that he/she was not good enough. This led to the family member sharing deeper, unshared feelings with God, like feelings of abandonment and loneliness. It is essential to realize that the primary purpose of this question is for the family member to learn how to share with God those feelings that most of us want to hide. This level of sharing fosters intimacy and trust.

QUESTION 4 often elicits a reaction from family members, especially those with a religious background, because of the part of Step 11 that says, "...praying *only* for knowledge of His will for us and courage to carry that out." Christianity and other faith traditions have a long history of intercessory prayers where the supplicant asks God to do something for someone else. A family member's prayer for their loved one's sobriety is intercessory. The 11th Step asks to limit prayer to just praying for God to share His will for us and then praying for God to give us the ability to do His will. The following may help guide discussions with the family members about the benefits of this approach to prayer when dealing with SUD in the family. The objective of the discussion is not to dissuade a family member from praying for other things but to provide the family member first with an understanding of the power of this approach to prayer. Second, guide the family's intercessory prayers by incorporating the principles of recovery.

- **GOD'S PLAN FOR MY LOVED ONE, NOT MINE.** Asking God for an outcome presupposes that the outcome is the best for the person and is also in God's plan. Eric and Joanne's early intercessory prayer for their loved one was for their daughter to be sober. There were several unspoken caveats to the prayer. The first was the timing for sobriety. They wanted their daughter to be sober immediately. The second was how she was to get sober. She was to get sober without an arrest record, without pain, without hurting Eric and Joanne, without a relapse, without hurting anyone else, and while graduating from high school and going directly to college. In other words, Eric and Joanne were not just asking God for their daughter's sobriety; they were telling God when and how they wanted Him to do it. As they continued in their recovery, Eric and Joanne's prayer became asking for God to grant their daughter sobriety in God's time and in God's way. Finally, their prayer became, "Please let our daughter seek God's will and pray for the courage to carry it out."

- **GOD'S PLAN FOR ME.** Whether other types of prayer are or are not a part of the family member's prayer life, incorporating praying for knowledge of God's will and the courage to do it is essential for several reasons. First, to move the family member's focus away from something they cannot control, their loved one's sobriety, to something they can control, themselves. Second, it shifts the family member's focus from their loved one to their Higher Power. This shift fosters two critical things. The first is letting go. It is hard for a family member to let go of someone they focus on. It is hard for a family member to let go of outcomes when they believe they can get the outcomes *they want* by asking God. Second, this shift changes the family members' focus from their relationship with their loved ones to their relationship with God.

EXAMINE YOUR MEDITATION

As in any good relationship, there is a time for talking and a time for listening. In meditation, we listen to God. This is often harder than it sounds. Our lives involve so much self-centered thought that forgetting ourselves and listening to our Higher Power can take a lot of practice.

QUESTION 1 asks what purpose meditation serves in a recovery program. AA Step 11 states the first purpose—"Sought through prayer and meditation to improve our conscious contact with God as we understand Him…" Conscious contact means we know God's presence and His reality throughout the day. What conscious contact looks like is having spontaneous conversations with God like you would with a friend. These are the kinds of conversations that lead to intimacy and trust. Second, meditation offers respite and rest. A period of meditation can be a time for living in the moment and enjoying the moment. It can be a period of rejuvenation to provide the resilience needed to face the next challenge in the day.

QUESTION 2 asks the family member to describe their meditation process. Many will not be able to answer the question because they do not meditate, either because they choose not to or do not know how to meditate. There are a couple of options when providing resources to aid in meditation. The first is mindfulness meditation, where the focus is getting quiet and living in and appreciating the moment. The second is scriptural based. An effective way to encourage meditation is to ask them to meditate briefly (5 minutes) and then gradually increase the time. Multiple Apps are helpful for this. "Simply Being" is an example of an app focusing on meditation. SoulTime™ is an example of an App that is Christian scripture-based.

QUESTION 3 is the hardest for family members because it asks how their Higher Power speaks to them. While praying or meditating, it is not unusual to have random thoughts come and go. When specifically praying for knowledge of God's will, the meditation period is listening for that guidance from God. One of the difficulties is separating random self-generated thoughts on what to do next from the advice that God is giving. This can be a very individualized response that can change as the family member progresses in recovery. One anonymous family member described his journey in this way:

Early in recovery, I struggled to separate my will from God's will. When faced with one of those tough questions (Do I enforce a hard boundary or let it slide?) I usually went with the one that gave me the this-is-the-right-answer feeling. I called it a bells and whistles carnival feeling. I thought that was God speaking to me. Well, I was wrong. The carnival feeling was me trying to convince myself that my easy way was the right way. When I went with the carnival feeling, things usually were worse. Once I found that out, all I had to do was to do the opposite of whatever gave me the carnival feeling. It worked.

Learning how God talks to a person is a skill that needs to be practiced. Writing a letter to God and then writing God's response to the letter—discussed in the next section—can help family members learn how God talks to them.

A Letter to God and God's Reply

Writing a letter to God and then writing God's response to the letter is a common exercise done on retreats and other settings. In the context of family member recovery, the tool uses both prayer and a form of meditation to help the family member gain clarity on an issue troubling them. The prayer is the letter to God. This is where the family member tells God all about what is bothering them, and then the family member may ask for relief or ask God to fix whatever is wrong. Encourage the family member to include his/her feelings about what is troubling him. "I feel so angry, guilty, and helpless over my daughter's relapse." Encourage the family member to include their feelings about God, especially if they are angry with God. "God, I am so angry with You. Why didn't you protect them from this relapse?" What the letter to God can accomplish:

- **BRINGS CLARITY TO THE ISSUE TROUBLING THE FAMILY MEMBER.** In writing the letter to God, the family member must describe the issue accurately. This accuracy often shows inconsistencies in the family member's understanding of the event. More importantly, writing may show that the family member's misery is not due to the loved one's actions but to the family member's character defects.

- **PROVIDES RELIEF.** Expressing the problem and moving the problem from just living in your head to living on paper can provide emotional relief. This relief often serves as the impetus to continue sharing our lives with God intimately and honestly.

- **PROVIDES PRACTICE IN IMPROVING THE FAMILY MEMBER'S CONSCIOUS CONTACT WITH GOD.** Writing a letter to God is a conscious effort to communicate with God. Providing one layer of separation assists those who have trouble talking to God. Instead of talking to God, they are writing a letter. In many instances, what a person finds challenging to say face-to-face, they can more easily communicate in writing.

Writing God's response to the letter seems like an odd task. Well, it is a strange task, but it has a purpose. First, the family member writing a letter from God enables the family member to take a step back and see what is occurring from a more detached perspective. In essence, the family member is asked to "act as if" they had lovingly detached from the situation. Often, family members can move from "acting as if" they had detached to detaching. One anonymous family member said, "When I wrote my second letter to my Higher Power, I could lovingly detach from the situation for the briefest moment. The relief I felt from detaching was overwhelming."

Second, writing the letter from God forces the family members to think about how their Higher Power would respond. Would it be an angry response? A rebuke-filled response? A loving response? A kind response? This kind of thinking clarifies the family member's perception of God so that they can identify any beliefs blocking their recovery. One of the most debilitating beliefs for a family member is that God is untrustworthy because it undermines the family member's ability to detach and let go. Recognizing they have this belief is the first of many steps in changing this belief.

Parting Thoughts on Strengthening a Relationship with a Higher Power

As demonstrated in the drum circle analogy in Chapter 5, our Higher Power is the basic beat of recovery. The family member's Higher Power and the Higher Power that they see in other family members provide:

- **THE INCENTIVE TO CHOOSE TO JOIN AND REMAIN IN THE PROGRAM.** Going to the first meeting is either an act of desperation or the result of an invitation. Usually, attending the first meeting results from desperation and invitation. Choosing to go back to a meeting is typically the result of the relief felt from meeting with people who understand. In drum circle terms, the relief is the result of the basic beat of the drum circle. The basic beat is God.

- **THE ABILITY TO UNCONDITIONALLY LOVE AND UNCONDITIONALLY ACCEPT PEOPLE.** The basic beat of the drum circle (God) allows disparate instruments and diverse rhythms to meld into one harmonious song that brings serenity, joy, and resilience. Part of learning to love and accept us.

- **THE ABILITY TO ACCEPT OUTCOMES AND LET GO OF OUR LOVED ONES.** Being aligned with the drum circle's basic beat allows one to accept others' decisions. The more the focus is on the basic beat (Higher Power), the more the power of God is felt.

- **THE ABILITY TO RECOVER FROM TRAGEDY.**

The development of a strong, trusting, intimate relationship with a Higher Power is the bedrock for recovery from SUD and especially for recovery from codependence. Building this relationship with a Higher Power is a personal process, often resulting from adversity. Adversity often catalyzes someone to strengthen their relationship with their Higher Power. The recovery coach must not short-circuit the work adversity is doing in a family member.

Writing a letter to and from God is best done with pen and paper. The tactile sensation of holding the pen and feeling the pen move across the paper engages more of the family member's senses. Looking at the writing itself—how the letters are formed, their size, and legibility—provides another expression of what happens inside the family member while writing the letter. It also gives the family members a visual means of expressing their feelings. These cues are helpful when the family member writes the letters but more helpful when the family member rereads the letter later.

CHAPTER 14

Moving from Non-recovery Beliefs to Recovery Beliefs

Much of the misery, anger, anxiety, and depression a family member feels is rooted in their non-recovery beliefs. The most common non-recovery belief is that addiction is a choice. This chapter aims to show how the event-Emotion-belief-feeling-action (EEBFA) process can first identify the non-recovery beliefs plaguing the family member and then facilitate the family member's adoption of recovery beliefs. The objectives of this chapter are to provide:

- An understanding of the EEBFA process.

- A methodology for assisting family members in identifying their codependent beliefs and the impact these beliefs have on their lives.

- A method to assist family members in transitioning from codependent beliefs to recovery beliefs.

This chapter starts with an explanation of the EEBFA process. Then, it discusses the non-recovery and recovery belief systems for family members in a way that gives a "head" and a "heart" understanding of these beliefs. The following section guides using Appendix N: Worksheet for the Event, Emotion, Belief, Feeling, Action Process to help family members understand how recovery and non-recovery beliefs impact their lives and their loved ones. EEBFA can help in changing belief systems by creating a desire to change.

The Event, Emotion, Belief, Feeling, and Action Process

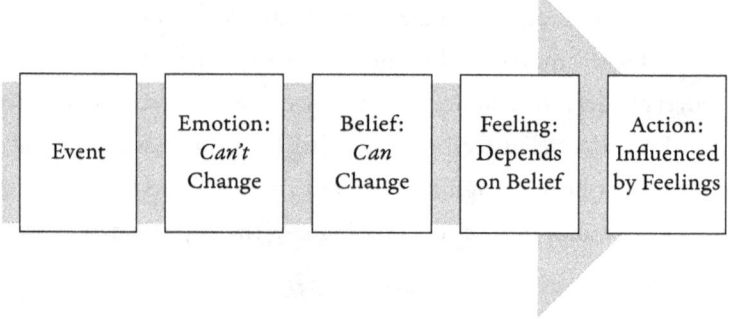

FIGURE 15. EVENT, EMOTION, BELIEF, FEELING, ACTION PROCESS

The EEBFA process is an adaptation of cognitive behavioral therapy (CBT). Aaron Beck developed CBT as a therapeutic intervention for many mental health issues that recognizes the causal link between beliefs and feelings. (Chand, Kuckel and Hueker 2024) *Figure 15* above illustrates the EEBFA process used in recovery circles to facilitate the adoption of recovery beliefs. The process starts with an initiating event. The event is a specific action or occurrence. For a family member, the event could be a loved one coming home drunk. The event causes an emotion. Emotions and feelings are similar, but they are not the same. In this model, emotion is the body's immediate response to the event. Emotions are hard-wired and occur immediately after the event. The purpose of an emotion is to ensure safety and survival (Delgado 2020, Hampton 2015, Shaver, et al. 1987). For example, a person is surprised (the emotion) when a stranger unexpectedly bumps into them (the event). The person did not choose to be surprised when the stranger bumped into them. The surprise was immediate and uncontrolled.

A person's belief about the event will determine the person's feelings. A feeling can last a long time—think about resentments. For example, if you believe the stranger bumped into you to cut in line, you might be angry and respond angrily. On the other hand, if you think they bumped into you as a pretext for meeting you, you might feel flattered and react in a calm, friendly manner. The same event and same emotion but different beliefs lead to different feelings and actions. Your brain uses your belief system, what you believe to be accurate, to assign meaning and feelings to the emotion and the event (Hampton 2015).

The last step in the process is the response to the event or action. It is important to note that feelings do not control actions; feelings only influence actions. Despite being angry at the line-cutter, you can choose to respond in a calm, polite manner. Since feelings do not dictate actions, feelings cannot justify one's actions. Feelings are responsible for much of the misery a family member feels. The family member's belief system is the only part of the emotion-to-feeling process they can control. A large part of recovery is changing our belief system when it comes to SUD and recovery.

Changing beliefs, especially long-held beliefs, is a mind-heart process. The first step is gaining an understanding of recovery beliefs. The second step is gaining real buy-in. The family member's progression usually starts with agreeing with some of the beliefs and disagreeing with others; continues with the family member believing the recovery beliefs but cannot implement them; and, finally, they are able to implement recovery beliefs. Be patient with family members and provide them with grace during this intervening period. The recovery coach needs to keep several things in mind about the family member during this process:

- Many of what we are calling codependent beliefs were valid and worked before their loved one became addicted and worked to raise their other children who did not have substance use issues. If their loved one is in the experimentation phase, the loved one can stop, and bailing them out may be appropriate. For some, using substances is just a phase, and they may stop of their own accord.

- Family members, friends, pastors, and sometimes physicians can reinforce non-recovery beliefs.

- Sometimes awful things do happen to their loved ones.

- Sometimes, family members, including parents/guardians, encouraged drug use.

The worksheet in Appendix N: Worksheet for the Event, Emotion, Belief, Feeling, Action Process on page 349, helps family members identify their non-recovery beliefs, understand the negative impact these beliefs have on the entire family, and experience the change when the non-recovery belief changes to a recovery belief. The worksheet then takes the family member through the EEBFA process with the non-recovery belief and then with the recovery belief. The worksheet has lists of non-recovery beliefs and recovery beliefs.

Non-Recovery and Recovery Beliefs

The non-recovery belief system makes recovery more difficult. The purpose of this section is to list common non-recovery beliefs and to provide insights to help understand the belief and the potential impact on the family member, the loved one, and the rest of the family. The following is a discussion of each of the codependent beliefs:

- **USING IS A LACK OF WILLPOWER. THEY COULD STOP IF THEY WANTED TO.** When discussing this belief with family members, it is important to remember that this is a true statement for loved ones who are in the experimentation (acquaintance) phase and the seeking (friendship) phase of substance use. It is less accurate for loved ones in the abuse/risky use (committed) phase and incorrect for loved ones in the addiction/dependence (enslaved) phase of SUD.

- **IT IS MY FAULT THAT MY LOVED ONE IS USING MIND-ALTERING SUBSTANCES. I CAUSED THIS BECAUSE I DID NOT PARENT CORRECTLY.** Parents/guardians and, to a lesser extent, other family members are telling family members either directly or indirectly that the loved one's SUD is a result of what the family member did wrong. Bad parenting, abusive parenting, no parenting, parents/guardians using, and parents/guardians encouraging drug use all enable SUD, but they do not cause it. The loved one still has the power of choice, and multiple factors contribute to SUD, including genetics. Parents/guardians may have enabled drug use, but they did not cause SUD. Similarly, and this is important, good parenting does not prevent SUD; it only enables sobriety.

- **I CAN FIX THIS. I CAN GET THEM TO STOP.** This is not an idle belief. This belief is based on the parent/guardian's experience with their loved one. Up to the point where SUD entered the family, parents/guardians have had success in correcting their children using the tools their parents taught them.

- **IT IS JUST A PHASE. I DO NOT NEED TO DO ANYTHING. THEY WILL SNAP OUT OF IT.** It is important to remember that sometimes, it is just a phase. If the loved one is in the experimentation (acquaintance) or seeking (friends) phase, they can choose to stop. However, if the family member is seeking help, the loved one is more than likely in the abuse/risky use (committed) or addiction/dependency (enslaved) stage of SUD. There is one other dynamic in the family member's belief that it is just a phase. Many parents/guardians used substances, sometimes extensively, when they were young, and they were able to stop using or scale back their substance use.

- **I CAN SAVE THEM.** This belief resembles the belief that the parent/guardian can fix it. For some, this belief is more destructive because saving a loved one is a more potent driver and can expand to all areas of the loved one's life. Saving can include bailing them out of jail, doing their homework, lying for them, and financially supporting them.

- **MY LOVED ONE NEEDS HELP. I DO NOT NEED HELP. I DO NOT NEED A RECOVERY PROGRAM.** This is the primary barrier to a family member getting into recovery. In a way, this is logical. If a loved one has cancer, the family member does not need chemotherapy. Unlike cancer, SUD is a family disease and affects the whole family. Codependency is not characterized as a disease, but it does lead to conditions that are diseases—depression, anxiety, stress, and stress-related physical and mental disorders. Like cancer and other diseases, the family needs new tools to help their loved one. The family learns to take precautions after their loved one has had radiation treatment or chemotherapy. Similarly, families dealing with SUD need new tools to cope with their loved one's illness.

- **I CAN CONTROL MY LOVED ONE'S BEHAVIOR.** This is related to some of the other beliefs. What sets this apart is the lengths a parent/guardian will often go to control their loved one. In one case, parents alarmed all windows and doors and took turns sleeping by the front door to prevent their daughter from disarming the alarm. The daughter just disabled the alarm on her bedroom window and left through the window. This is a self-defeating belief, especially when setting and enforcing boundaries. This belief turns boundaries into punishments, with the parents looking for the consequence that will punish the loved one the most.

- **I CAN GUILT AND SHAME THEM INTO DOING WHAT I WANT THEM TO DO.** This is a destructive belief because of the shame and guilt the loved one already feels. As with each of the beliefs that deal with controlling, each time the parent/guardian fails to control the loved one, anger, resentment, and despair build. Despair is the most destructive of these because it pushes the family member further into their codependency and further away from recovery.

- **HOW CAN THEY DO THIS TO ME AFTER ALL I HAVE DONE FOR THEM?** It is common for a family member to believe that the loved one is using substances to hurt them. There is ample evidence to support this belief. The loved one will blame the family member. The loved one will say they use substances because of the family member. The loved one will steal and destroy property. Friends and family members who do not understand addiction reinforce this when they tell the parent/guardian: "How can you let him get away with that?" "If he were my child, I would never let that happen." "I cannot believe she is so mean to you." These statements place the parent/guardian in the role of a victim. Make no mistake, the loved one is hurting the family, but the disease of SUD is the motivation behind the actions, not the loved one's desire to hurt the family.

- **I WILL BAIL THEM OUT AGAIN TO GET THEM ON THE RIGHT TRACK. THEN THINGS WILL BE OKAY.** This is the "fresh start" cure. The underlying belief is that the loved one's substance use is because of all the trouble the loved one is in; getting them out of trouble relieves the stress, which leads to them stopping or at least controlling their substance use. For a loved one with SUD, bailing them out prevents the loved one from feeling the consequences of their drug use. Providing bail has other negative impacts. First, it denies the loved one the opportunity to fix the problem themselves so the loved one can feel the pride of working through adversity. Second, it sets the expectation that the family will always provide bail for the loved one. Third, it places the loved one squarely in the position of being a victim.

- **LETTING GO AND DETACHING ARE THE SAME AS GIVING UP.** This is a common, often firmly held belief early in the family member's recovery. In general, it is due to misunderstanding the recovery meaning of letting go and detaching. Letting go and detaching are not giving up but adopting approaches that have proven effective in dealing with SUD.

- **MY LOVED ONE CANNOT RECOVER WITHOUT MY HELP.** The primary fallacy in this belief is that the loved one must have the family member's help to recover. The loved one can recover with or without a family member's help. If the help the family member provides is codependent—bailing them out, lying for them, nagging, and shaming—the family member is enabling the continuance of the disease. Genuine concern for the loved one drives the family member's powerful desire to help. This drive is amplified by the family member's incorrect belief that the loved one is unable to recover without the family member intervening.

There are other less healthy drivers behind this belief. First is the need to be needed. Second and less common is the desire to be the person that saved the loved one. An anonymous family member said,

> I wanted to be the one that saved my child. I used to imagine my daughter coming up to me later in life and saying, "Dad, thank you for my sobriety. Remember the discussion on what my life could be like if I stopped using drugs? That was the moment that turned my life around." Now, I know it was selfish, but at the time, I was desperate for something to give me hope.

- **IF I LOVE THEM, I SHOULD TRUST THEM. IF I LOVE THEM, I SHOULD LIKE THEM.** This program is a program of unconditional love and not unconditional trust or unconditional like. The false belief that loving someone means liking and trusting them can create anguish in a family member in three ways. First, the family member may believe they must trust their loved one because the family member loves the loved one. A person with SUD is not trustworthy. Trusting the loved one before he is trustworthy enables the continuance of the disease and leads to family member resentment when the loved one betrays this trust. Second, a family member may question their love for the person with SUD because the family member does not trust nor like the loved one. A parent/guardian believing they do not love his child can be a source of misery and anguish.

- "I CAN LOVE THEM OUT OF THIS DISEASE. IF I LOVE THEM ENOUGH, THEY WILL QUIT." ANONYMOUS FAMILY GROUP MEMBER. The type of love the family group member referred to was "nice" love—giving the loved one everything they wanted. A loved one with SUD wants whatever they need to continue using. This belief also has the notion that the family member can do something to make the loved one quit using substances.

- I AM RESPONSIBLE FOR OUTCOMES. This common belief is reinforced in almost every aspect of life. This has already been discussed in detail above.

- GOD'S PLAN IS NOT WORKING, SO I WILL TAKE OVER. This belief can be stated more plainly: "God is not doing what I want Him to do. God is wrong. I am right, and I will do it my way." This belief is birthed in love, frustration, fear, shame, and guilt. The family member loves the afflicted person and cannot bear to see the loved one suffer and cannot bear their own suffering. The chronic, relapsing nature of SUD and the apparent lack of progress builds frustration and fear, especially when the family member is being asked to "Let go and let God."

Recovery beliefs are the core beliefs that foster recovery from codependency and addiction. This section discusses fundamental beliefs that can help a family member recover from codependence.

- **SUD IS A DISEASE.** This is the fundamental belief that allows responding versus reacting. It also is the basis for each of the remaining beliefs. The addiction process started with a choice—the choice to use. Roughly 10% of the using population will become addicted and will lose the power of choice (McLellan 2017). For the 10%, using is no longer fun, but they need to use substances to feel normal. At this point, it is a disease just like diabetes and cancer.

- **SUD AFFECTS THE WHOLE FAMILY; THE ENTIRE FAMILY NEEDS HELP.** This belief means that the whole family needs recovery. Sometimes, it is difficult for a family member to realize that SUD is affecting them and that they need help. The discussion of family roles in Chapter 2, Substance Use Disorder, Codependency, and Family Roles, is one method to help family members understand the impact of SUD on themselves and the rest of their family. It is difficult for a family member to accept this belief if they are in Stage 1 Codependency. In this stage, the family member believes the loved one's issues are like the issues the family has overcome before. The family member does not believe there is a problem. In Stage 2, the family is noticing detrimental changes in the loved one that place the family in a state of increased stress. The family may or may not be aware that it needs help. In Stages 3 and 4, it is increasingly clear that the family needs help.

- **THE 3 C'S.** You did not cause the disease, you cannot control the disease, and you cannot cure the disease. Believing the first "C" requires the family member to think that addiction is a disease. It is a disease that starts with a choice, the choice to use substances, but other diseases also begin with a choice. Tobacco-induced lung cancer, Type II diabetes, and cholesterol-related heart and artery diseases all start with the same choice many people make, but not all contract the disease. Everyone who smokes does not get lung cancer. Everyone who eats sweets does not contract Type II diabetes. Everyone who has a high-cholesterol diet does not contract heart disease. Genetics and other environmental factors beyond our control determine, in concert, whether the person contracts the disease.

Internalizing the next two "C's" is usually a slow process that involves meetings, appointments, and activities (having fun). Going to activities and having fun to foster these beliefs might seem surprising because the relationship is not apparent. Activities and having fun provide the family member a respite from the overwhelming fear that drives the need to control. Fear that something awful will happen to their loved one—the selfish fear of what the terrible event will do to the family member. The family member gets to experience the joy of not having the desperate need to cure and control.

- **RECOVERY CANNOT BE DONE ALONE; HOWEVER, EACH PERSON IS RESPONSIBLE FOR THEIR OWN RECOVERY.** An unwillingness to attend support group meetings, go to appointments, and get a sponsor is fostered by the family member's belief that they can and should deal with the addiction in their family by themselves. This belief is often unintentionally reinforced by the warning that one needs to work on their own program. It helps to portray meetings, appointments, and sponsorship as methodologies to learn the tools the family member needs to enable his own recovery and to stop enabling their loved one's drug use. The family member is responsible for understanding these tools, building the support network needed to use them effectively, and using them in a manner that is appropriate for the family member and their family. You cannot work someone else's program for them.

- **ENABLING A LOVED ONE'S SOBRIETY MEANS ALLOWING THEM TO FEEL THE NATURAL CONSEQUENCES OF THEIR SUBSTANCE USE.** Allowing a loved one to feel the natural consequences of their substance use is difficult and very necessary, especially if the loved one is in the addicted (enslaved) phase of substance use. Eric Daxon says, "I have never heard a loved one say they got sober because their parents were nice. I have heard quite a few say sobriety occurred after their parents started setting and enforcing boundaries." Be patient with family members. More than likely, the first time a family member hears this, they will think the worst—overdose, jail, killed, trafficked, etc. Hearing this belief in meetings, from their sponsor, and most importantly, hearing it from sober loved ones facilitates the adoption of this belief.

- **THIS IS A PROGRAM OF UNCONDITIONAL LOVE, NOT UNCONDITIONAL TRUST NOR UNCONDITIONAL LIKE.** Going over the Greek words for love found in Chapter 5 will help clarify what unconditional love means. It is agape love, which is choosing to love someone simply because of their humanity, simply because God loves them. Storge is the love family members have for one another. Storge is an excellent example because all family members have been angry with each other; all families have a member they do not trust. Storge is still there despite the anger and distrust.

- **LETTING GO AND DETACHING FOSTER RECOVERY IN YOU AND YOUR LOVED ONE.** One phrase common in recovery is, "Let go and let God." Letting go does not mean doing nothing. It advocates letting go of the things you cannot control so you can concentrate on the things you can control, like working on a recovery program. Often, family members focus on controlling things they cannot control (e.g., their loved one's sobriety) so much that they have no time to do what they can control—their own recovery.

Detaching is another problematic concept because it sounds uncaring and counterintuitive; however, detaching from a loved one with SUD is a kind and loving thing to do. In simplest terms, detaching means the family member will not allow their loved one's choices to ruin the family member's life. Detaching with love means still mourning the loved one's bad choices, but their choices will not destroy the family member. Detaching also means respecting the loved one's ability to choose while exercising our ability to choose. The critical part about detaching is when the loved one is sober; the loved one has a happy, healthy family member to return to.

I CAN CONTROL ONLY WHAT I SAY, WHAT I DO, WHAT I THINK, WHAT I BELIEVE, AND HOW I FEEL.[20] This belief is vital to family member recovery from codependency because it fosters letting go of outcomes and prompts the family member to focus on what they can change—themselves. For most people, the ability to control thoughts and feelings is a new concept. We cannot control all the thoughts that enter our minds. However, we always control which thoughts we choose to dwell on. Many believe that feelings just are, and they occur in response to a stimulus. The EEBFA model discussed earlier

---

20 There are some categories of feelings that we cannot control. Feelings associated with being sick, and feelings associated with mental illness are beyond our ability to control without professional help.

in this chapter shows the link between our feelings, the thoughts we dwell on, and the beliefs we choose to hold.

- **GOD'S PLAN AND NOT MY PLAN.** Adopting this belief usually results from working a diligent program—attending meetings, sponsors, activities, and appointments. The recovery coach can assist by first meeting and accepting the family members where they are. If the family member does not have a Higher Power, work with them on their Higher Power. The coach can share his journey with God. Eric Daxon describes how a recovery coach helped him with this belief.

> It was a simple yet powerful thing the recovery coach did. She told me to borrow her Higher Power and act as if I believed God had a plan for me and my loved one when things got tough. It worked. I was able to experience the relief that this letting go offered. When I hit my bottom, it was second nature for me to turn to God.

Using Appendix N: Worksheet for the Event, Emotion, Belief, Feeling, Action Process

The purpose of this worksheet is to highlight the importance of recovery beliefs in relieving the misery a family member experiences when SUD is in the family. The worksheet does this by distinguishing between emotions—which cannot be changed—and feelings—which can be changed if the family member changes their beliefs from non-recovery to recovery beliefs. The worksheet has examples of both. The approach is to take the family member through a mental process of comparing their imagined response to an event with a non-recovery belief (e.g., SUD is not a disease) and their imagined response if they changed to a recovery belief (e.g., SUD is a disease).

QUESTION 1 asks the family member to list what the loved one did to cause harm to the family member and the entire family. This is an opportunity for the recovery coach to gain a fuller understanding of the dynamics in the family, the phase of codependency the family member is in, as well as the stage of SUD for the loved one. In guiding the family member through this question, be aware of any resentments the family member had before SUD came into the family. These resentments fuel non-recovery beliefs and counterproductive responses. If the resentments are severe enough, the family member may need to do a specific inventory of that resentment.

QUESTION 2 asks the family member to select the three most notable events. When discussing these, asking the family member what sets these events apart is helpful. This will give the recovery coach a better understanding of the beliefs contributing to the hurt or the non-recovery response. It also allows the family member to think critically about the event again.

QUESTION 3 asks the family member to pick one of the three events and describe it in enough detail that someone else could understand how the event hurt the family member. This is a time to ask questions that can reveal the beliefs operating in the event. It is common for a family member to deny having any non-recovery beliefs. This can be because the family member is in denial, is embarrassed to admit a non-recovery belief, is trying to impress the recovery coach, or is trying to defend their response to the loved one.

QUESTION 4 asks the family members to identify their emotions immediately following the event. The exercise uses five standard emotions—love, joy, anger, sadness, fear, and surprise.

QUESTION 5 asks the family member to identify the feeling or what they felt after the initial emotion subsided. Some examples will help the family members understand. The emotion associated with smelling alcohol on the loved one's breath could be sadness or surprise, followed by anger and despair. The emotions of anger and hopelessness may linger, which turns them into feelings.

QUESTION 6 asks the family member to identify what the family member did in response to the event. Dwell on this question with the family member. Ask them how they felt after they responded. Ask them how things turned out with the loved one, family members, and family. The more discussions about the family members' responses, the better the family members and the recovery coach can identify the family members' beliefs.

QUESTION 7 asks about the family member's beliefs. The first step in the recovery coach's discussions with the family member is to ensure the beliefs the family member selected are accurate. Choosing a belief incongruent with the family member's story can be due to a lack of understanding, denial, minimization, or several other reasons.

QUESTION 8 asks the family member to change the non-recovery belief to a recovery belief and replay the event. This is a suitable time for the recovery coach to share their personal experience of how the recovery coach's life changed and how the family changed when the recovery coach adopted recovery beliefs in their head and heart.

QUESTION 9 asks the family member which belief, non-recovery or recovery, they think would be more effective for her, the loved one, and the rest of the family.

Parting Thoughts on Event, Emotion, Belief, Feeling, Action

The EEBFA process gives the family member a better "head-understanding" of recovery beliefs and starts giving them a "heart-understanding" of recovery beliefs. The process of believing a belief and being able to act in accordance with that belief is a slow one that includes relapse. Framing the transformation process in this way will help relieve the shame and guilt that comes with a relapse. It is also important that the recovery coach has a head and heart-understanding of the role relapse plays in a family member's process of transforming their beliefs. This understanding helps alleviate a recovery coach's frustration toward a family member who is not acting on a belief.

This can be a challenging exercise if the family member is in Stage 1 Codependency or Stage 4, this can be a challenging exercise because of the denial that may exist in Stage 1 and the depression that may exist in Stage 4. If nothing else, the family member will gain the head knowledge of recovery beliefs, which is the first step in belief transformation.

One facilitator of belief change is seeing that others hold and act on recovery beliefs. As mentioned in Chapter 9, Barriers to Recovery, meetings, working with a sponsor, and attending activities provide opportunities to hear about other's experiences with changing their beliefs. This also allows the family member to witness the change in group members' lives. Seeing people in dire straits having joy in their lives and knowing what to do in situations that used to "baffle" them is powerful proof that recovery beliefs work.

The EEBFA can lead to the false belief that feelings will dictate actions. Statements like, "My anger drove me to hit him" are wrong. The correct way to make that statement is, "I was angry, and I *chose* to hit him." Feelings influence responses, but feelings do not dictate responses. As people in recovery often say, "Feelings are not facts." Decisions need to be based on facts. In every situation, recovery calls on us to always do the next right thing. Feelings influence actions, but feelings never justify actions.

CHAPTER 15

Overcoming Guilt and Shame

A common saying in recovery circles is, "Secrets keep you sick." This is especially true if the secrets are hidden actions that are still causing guilt and, worse yet, shame. What stays in the dark often festers in the dark. Guilt and shame-driven secrets can create a walled-off area in a person's personality in which a person tries to keep others out, tries to keep themselves out, and even tries to keep their Higher Power from knowing. The latter is a *non-sequitur* because most believe their Higher Power is all-knowing, yet the erroneous belief remains. The original writers of the 12 Steps knew this, and that is why the 5th Step requires admitting our wrongs "...*to God*, to ourselves, and to another human being..." (Alcoholics Anonymous 2019). It is not surprising that the primary method for dealing with both shame and guilt is working the 12 Steps with a sponsor. The purpose of this chapter is to suggest tools that can assist in this process. Specifically, the objectives of this chapter are to:

- Provide an intellectual and emotional understanding of a family member's guilt and shame.

- Provide tools for a recovery coach to use to aid a family member in working through shame and guilt.

As discussed, the primary tool is working the 12 Steps with a sponsor. This chapter describes three tools a recovery coach can use to help a family member work through guilt/shame. The first tool is education, which specifically targets guilt and shame. In addition to defining guilt and shame, this section discusses free will and our inability to control outcomes. Not understanding these two concepts can generate misplaced guilt/shame in all family members, especially parents/guardians.

The second tool is a guilt-specific inventory in Appendix O: Guilt and Shame Inventory on page 355. This inventory aims to help the family member identify and critically assess the guilt/shame-producing event so the family member can take appropriate action to resolve the guilt or shame blocking their recovery. The third tool guides the discussion when the family member and the recovery coach review the family member's inventory.

The coach must consider several issues when using this tool. First, the guilt inventory is not a replacement for working the 12 Steps but an augmentation designed to help someone who is stuck in their recovery because of guilt/shame. Second, the coach must know the family member's codependency stage. If the family member is in Stage 4 Codependency, these tools might not be practical until the family member receives a higher level of care. Third, the guilt/shame may come from traumatic experiences that may also require a higher level of care than a recovery coach can provide. Examples of these include inflicting or receiving severe childhood trauma; serious suicidal ideation or suicide attempts; commission of or being the victim of extreme abuse; commission of or being the victim of a serious crime; and actions related to severe mental illnesses like PTSD and schizophrenia.

Guilt/Shame Education

Concepts addressed in this section include guilt/shame, free will, and control (or lack thereof) of outcomes. These topics are interrelated because most of the family members' unjustified guilt/shame comes from not understanding free will and not understanding the relationship between family members' actions and the outcomes.

WHAT ARE GUILT AND SHAME?

First, both guilt and shame are feelings. With guilt, the belief is, "I did something wrong." Guilt is a healthy feeling because it helps identify right from wrong. It is usually act specific: "I stole from the corner store, and I feel guilty." Guilt is also a motivator to make amends for the harm done. A healthy sense of guilt fosters recovery. Unresolved guilt, or a guilt that lingers, is harmful because it can turn into shame or deep resentment.

The same is not valid for shame. The belief with shame is not "I did something wrong." With shame, the belief is, "I am bad," "I am unlovable," "I am not worthy," or "I am not likable." The worst manifestation of shame is when the family member believes, "I am evil." Shame hinders recovery because it causes people to turn inward, away from others and their Higher Power. It can create a dark place that hinders or even blocks recovery.

Long-held guilt/shame can fall into three categories. The first is guilt or shame based on the act's inherent wrongness, whether the outcome is good or bad. Stealing, murder, adultery, lying with malicious intent, using illegal drugs, distributing illicit drugs, and gossiping are examples of inherently wrong actions. Regardless of the outcome, guilt or shame still exists because the acts are inherently wrong. The second is outcomes-based guilt/shame. This is guilt based on the result of an action, whether the action was right or wrong. An example is a parent feeling guilty because the loved one ran away after the parent enforced a boundary. The third is guilt/shame generated by false beliefs. The primary guilt/shame-inducing false beliefs are the inverse of the 3 C's, "I cause the addiction. I can control the addiction. I can cure the addiction."

FREE WILL

Family members, especially parents/guardians, often have difficulty understanding the implications of free will for their children. Many believe that if a parent/guardian raises a child correctly, they will become a good adult who will always do right and make good choices. Many also believe that if the child does wrong and makes poor choices, it is because of bad parenting. These two false beliefs are the source of a great deal of unwarranted grief and shame for parents/guardians. Good parenting enables a child to make good choices; it does not guarantee that the child will make good choices. The child still has the power to choose. Eric tells a story that often helps parents/guardians understand how good parenting can result in a child making bad choices. Here is Eric's story:

> Joanne and I heard a sermon in a large church where the pastor went through a biblical list of how a parent should raise a child. The pastor did not imply but said that if a child is on the wrong path, the parents did not do one of the things on his biblical list. To illustrate his point, the pastor had his sons on stage with him and said words to the effect, "I did all these things, and all of my sons choose to be pastors of their own free will." In short, the pastor said his good parenting led to his children doing well.
>
> I was fuming when I heard this and drafted an email to the pastor about the story of Adam, Eve, Cain, and Abel. Here is the gist of my email, "God, the perfect father, raised Adam and Eve. What did Adam and Eve do? They broke one of only two rules God gave Adam and Eve. Cain and Abel were raised by parents whom the perfect father taught. What did Cain do? Cain murdered Abel. Despite "perfect parenting," Adam, Eve, and Cain chose to do evil because God gave us all free will.

He gave us the ability to choose freely. The same is true for us and our children."

Unfortunately, the pastor did not respond to the email. As a side note, Joanne and I were at a service led by his oldest son. The oldest son said that before he was a pastor, he was an engineer working at an engineering firm and loved it. The oldest son became a pastor because his dad kept badgering him.

WE DO NOT CONTROL OUTCOMES

This section addresses guilt or shame generated by believing someone can control outcomes. Outcomes-based guilt or shame is often based on the belief that the person's action or inaction was solely responsible for the negative outcome.

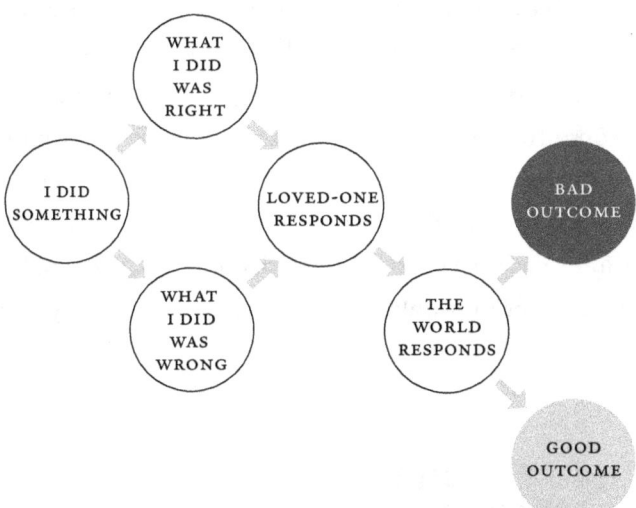

FIGURE 16. NOTIONAL RELATIONSHIP BETWEEN DOING RIGHT OR WRONG THING AND OUTCOMES

Figure 16, on the previous page, shows a notional diagram of the relationship between a family member's action affecting a loved one and the uncontrollable factors influencing the outcome. The process is the same whether what the family member did was right or wrong. The loved one will respond to that act in either a healthy or unhealthy way. The family member cannot control the loved one's response. Then, forces beyond the control of the family member or the loved one will respond to the actions of the family member and the loved one. The outcome, good or bad, is the final link in the chain.

Getting a job promotion is a simple example of the process outlined in *Figure 16*. A person can do everything they need to do to get the promotion. They can work hard, obtain the required training, go the extra mile, surpass all their goals, and be a team player. They can do all the right things and still not receive the promotion because of factors beyond their control. For example, the company might go out of business. There may be six equally qualified candidates for one position. An unexpected downturn could result in eliminating the position they were seeking. The boss may hire someone else as a favor to a close friend. The person did everything they could do to deserve the promotion, but events beyond the person's control resulted in a bad outcome—no promotion.

We cannot control outcomes, but we can influence them. In the promotion example above, taking all the actions needed to deserve the promotion puts the person in a position to get the promotion. The harder the person worked, the more they influenced the selection authority to promote them. Refusing to prepare for a promotion would affect the selection authority to choose someone else.

NON-RECOVERY BELIEFS GENERATE GUILT/SHAME

Non-recovery beliefs like the 3 C's are the source of many undeserved guilty feelings. Substituting a recovery belief for a non-recovery belief can transform what the family member believes is a bad outcome into a good outcome. For example, the police arresting a loved one for DUI is a good outcome if the family member understands both the nature of the disease of SUD and the need for the loved one to feel the consequences of their substance use. The loved one getting arrested is a bad outcome if the family member still believes protecting the loved one at all costs is the right thing to do. The EEBFA tool discussed in Chapter 14 can help identify and transform the non-recovery beliefs into recovery beliefs.

Using Appendix O: Guilt and Shame Inventory

The purpose of the worksheet in Appendix O: Guilt and Shame Inventory is to help a family member accomplish three tasks. First, identify the event(s) generating the guilt or shame that is blocking their recovery. Second, fully understand the source of the guilt/shame. Third, develop a plan to resolve the guilt/shame that is blocking their recovery.

The first part of this section (Illustrative Family Member Stories) has family member stories the authors will use to aid in discussing the questions in the guilt/shame inventory. The stories are either from one of the authors or the author's work with family members. James, Sebastian, Carol, and Meg are fictitious names for family members who worked with the authors.

The second part of this section (Explanation of the Questions in Appendix O: Guilt and Shame Inventory) provides the recovery coach with a more detailed explanation of the questions in Appendix O. The third part of this section (Discussing Guilt/Shame Inventory Answers with the Family Member) provides guidance on how the recovery coach can use the action-outcome process shown *Figure 16* to help the family member identify the specific cause of their guilt/shame. Once the family member identifies the cause, the recovery coach can assist the family member to do the "next right thing" to resolve the often debilitating feelings of guilt or shame.

ILLUSTRATIVE FAMILY MEMBER STORIES

Family member stories illustrate one or more aspects of the concepts discussed in this chapter. James, Sebastian, Carol, and Meg are fictitious names for real people who worked with the authors. Each of these worked hard to recover from codependency or SUD and are living full, productive lives.

Eric's Story

Eric's middle school (yes, middle school) guilt/shame story is an example of the need for specificity when describing the guilt/shame-generating events. Dave P. embarrassed Eric in front of several classmates. Eric felt ashamed, and the shame turned into a strong resentment that Eric held onto for over 30 years. Naturally, Dave P. was on Eric's inventory. Eric's sponsor asked him to think carefully about the encounter, describe what happened, and remember his feelings.

As Eric started writing, he wondered why Dave P.'s insult stuck with him like it did. People insulted Eric before this, and people insulted Eric after this, but for some reason, Dave P.'s insult was the one that Eric held on to. When Eric reexamined the event, he remembered Dave taunting him. Eric also remembered something that he had forgotten. Eric responded to Dave's taunt, but it was a "lame" response because Eric was afraid of Dave. Dave was a big guy. In talking about this, Eric realized that it was not the insult that generated the shame. The shame came because middle-school Eric held the false belief that his fear of Dave meant he was a coward. Eric also realized that his actions demonstrated that he was brave. He responded to Dave's taunt despite his fear.

James' Story

James felt guilt and shame over an incident that happened when his daughter (his loved one) was in middle school. James loved to run alone. It was his favorite pastime because not only did James enjoy the exercise, but he enjoyed the solitude. As he was preparing to leave, his daughter asked James if she could run with him. James said, "No." James' excuse was that his daughter was slow, and he wanted to go on a long, fast run. James really said no because he wanted to be alone. James tried to justify his "no" to himself, but he knew he was just being selfish. He felt guilty about the "no."

When his daughter's SUD bloomed, James' guilt over saying "no" turned into shame. James came to believe that his "no" was the start of his daughter's addiction. This belief came about because James believed what people were telling him: His daughter's addiction was James' fault. As James put it:

> When my daughter's drug use flared, I was desperate to find a cause for her using drugs. Many around me obliged me by telling me drug use was the parent's fault. The selfish "no" started to take on increased significance, and the 'no' turned into "I caused my daughter's addiction because I did not spend time with her." I did not want anyone to know that I caused my daughter's addiction, so I kept it to myself.
>
> I started fantasizing what it would be like if I said "yes" to the run. I imagined the "yes" turning into regular father-daughter runs that deepened into the type of relationship that would have stopped my daughter from using. I was guilty over the "no." I was remorseful over the relationship that never happened because of the "no." I was guilty over my daughter's resulting addiction. The guilt rapidly turned into shame. I was a bad dad. This false belief drove my early denial. It also drove my early hesitancy to embrace the program. I was a bad dad who did not deserve happiness. This also made it hard for me to enforce the tough, necessary boundaries. How could I be "mean" to my daughter if I caused it?

Sebastian's Story

Sebastian had two sons, and he and they had drug use issues. In a men's meeting, Sebastian admitted that he used to coach his sons on how to use drugs—what drug combinations were good and which ones to avoid. Sebastian was able to stop using drugs and alcohol eventually, but his sons were not. Sebastian sought help when one of his son's drug use (Joe) became entirely out of control. Sebastian was convinced that his coaching was the reason Joe became a drug addict.

Carol's Story

Carol was a recently divorced mom with two children. Her marriage was rocky, and the divorce was inevitable. Like most single moms, Carol worked hard all day and then came home to two children who needed her complete attention. One night, she came home extremely tired. Her youngest child, Jason, was crying and needed his diaper changed. Carol knew this but was fatigued, so she fell onto her bed and slept.

Years later, Jason developed severe SUD, and Carol came for help. Carol and her coach worked on boundaries. Carol knew boundaries, even the tough ones, were a part of Jason's recovery. Jason got into trouble and wanted Carol to post bail for him. Carol knew it was wrong but bailed Jason out anyway. In discussions with her coach, Carol said she had to bail him out because she neglected Jason in the past. When the coach asked how she failed Jason, Carol told the story of not changing Jason's diaper.

Meg's Story

Meg was a family group member who had a 16-year-old son, Josh, with severe SUD. Josh was driving high and totaled his truck. He was distraught, apologetic, and promised to enter recovery. Josh asked Meg to replace his truck so he could get to work. Meg believed him, wanted Josh to keep his job, and agreed to give him a "fresh start" by replacing his truck. Meg felt the "fresh start" worked because Josh was sober for a couple of months; then, he relapsed and totaled another truck. Meg gave Josh another "fresh start" and bought him another truck. Again, he was driving under the influence and totaled this truck. Josh wrecked six trucks over two years, and Meg replaced each of the six because, in part, Meg believed the "first fresh" start worked.

Remember that Meg was a good, hard-working woman trying her best to enable her son to succeed. She knew that Josh needed to feel the consequences of driving under the influence. She also remembered the importance of her first job to becoming financially independent and living a comfortable life. She wanted the same for her son. The fear she felt over her son being jobless was the primary reason she could not allow her son to be without a vehicle. I need to say that again. She lacked the ability. Her Higher Power had not yet given her the ability to really let go of her son. Please remember this and treat family members with the same kindness and compassion as you might for a substance user in trouble.

EXPLANATION OF THE QUESTIONS IN APPENDIX O: GUILT AND SHAME INVENTORY

The first step in helping a family member work through guilt/shame is understanding the event(s) that triggered the guilt/shame. The questions in Appendix O provide the family member with a tool to describe the guilt/shame-producing event or action accurately.

QUESTION 1 in the inventory asks the family member to list the past or current events that generate feelings of guilt or shame. This is just a listing of the events. Encourage the family member to answer this question as briefly as possible. Succinctness provides the clarity needed to identify the specific event generating guilt and shame. For Eric, being embarrassed by Dave P. was the event. For James, the event was saying "No" when his daughter asked to go on a run with him. For Sebastian, the event was teaching his sons how to use drugs. For Carol, the event was not changing her son's dirty diaper. If the family member does not give a brief answer, continue to probe until the family member gets to the actual event generating the guilt. Meg's guilt was a little different. Her guilt stemmed from the belief that she was responsible for her son's success.

QUESTION 2 asks the family member to factually describe the event without ascribing blame and include the information requested by the sub-questions. QUESTION 2A asks for a detailed description of what happened at each event. This is, as the folks on Dragnet would say, "Just the facts, Ma'am." Sometimes, just going through the event's facts will resolve guilt and shame, as in Eric's case. Eric's shame was the false belief that he was a coward. Two things contributed to the staying power of Eric's shame. First, in middle school, Eric had a false belief about cowardice; he equated fear with being a coward. Second, older Eric did not remember responding to Dave's insult. Older Eric knew that acting despite being afraid was courage and not cowardice. Writing about the event in detail allowed Eric to put these puzzle pieces together. Eric's next step was to forgive himself for holding onto a false, hurtful memory for so long.

QUESTION 2B asks the family member to focus on what the family member did that was the source of the guilt/shame and determine if the act was wrong. Whether the act was right or wrong, the question further asks if the act caused harm. In Eric's case, neither he nor Dave P. did anything inherently wrong. Dave embarrassed Eric, and Eric gave a less-than-adequate retort. James did nothing inherently wrong when he said no to his daughter coming with him on the run. James's "no" is not what generated the guilt James felt. It was James' real motivation for saying no, selfishness, that led to James' lasting guilt.

In Sebastian's case, his actions were inherently wrong, but the feelings of guilt did not manifest until Sebastian entered recovery. Giving his sons advice on what drugs to use, teaching them how to use them, and providing them with drugs were all inherently wrong. At the time, Sebastian did not believe what he was doing was wrong because, first, Sebastian was using illegal drugs. Second, his motivation was his sons' safety. Sebastion wanted to make sure his sons' drug use did not harm them. When Sebastian entered recovery, his beliefs about illegal drug use changed from acceptance to understanding its inherent wrongness.

In Carol's case, not changing Jason's diaper was symbolic of what she believed was her neglect of Jason throughout his life. She attributed Jason's drug use to her neglect. Carol did not neglect Jason any more than most parents neglect their children. A deeper dive into Carol's story revealed that she viewed not giving Jason what he wanted (vs. needed) as neglect.

Meg still believed that replacing her son's wrecked trucks was the right thing to do even though she knew it was enabling. Like the person with SUD, sometimes the family member continues in spite of the consequences.

The intent of QUESTION 2C is to help the family member focus on the harm caused by the act to identify the harm and who the act harmed. In most instances, the harm and the person causing the harm are readily identifiable. This is not always the case. In Eric's case, the overt act of Dave P. insulting Eric did not cause Eric's long-term guilt. The source of Eric's guilt/shame was the false belief that he was a coward because he felt fear. Dave P. was a part of Eric's first and second inventory, but the resentment and the guilt remained until Eric identified the natural source of the guilt.

QUESTION 3 asks the family member to review what they wrote in QUESTION 2 and compare it to the memory fueling the guilt/shame identified in QUESTION 1. The memory of an event that people carry daily is sometimes inaccurate or incomplete. Often, the inaccuracies or the left-out parts generate guilt or shame. The day-to-day memory led the family member to add the event in QUESTION 1. QUESTION 2 asks the family member to go past the everyday memory and remember the event. There are often differences, and these differences can be significant. The root cause of the resentment that plagued Eric for 30 years was a false belief that he was a coward. Carefully reexamining the event helped Eric identify the false belief driving the shame and resentment. In James' story, he believed that saying "no" to his daughter was a major cause of her drug addiction. Carol thought that not changing her son's dirty diaper meant she neglected him for his entire life. This was not the case.

The last sub-bullet in QUESTION 3 asks about barriers to doing the next right thing—amends or forgiving. The barriers will likely be one of those listed in Chapter 9, Barriers to Recovery. Use the guidance in Chapter 9 to develop a way ahead.

DISCUSSING GUILT/SHAME INVENTORY ANSWERS WITH THE FAMILY MEMBER

The guilt/shame inventory aims to start the guilt/shame mitigation process by asking the family member to recall, think about, and write down the critical components of their guilt/shame. The next step is for the family member to discuss their answers with their recovery coach. This section provides a framework for the recovery coach to use when talking to the family member about the worksheet. The framework is based on the steps between action and outcome, as shown in *Figure 16* above.

Is the Action Right or Wrong?

In outcomes-based thinking, an action is right or wrong, depending on the outcome. The first step in helping a family member address guilt/shame based on outcomes is determining whether the action taken by the family member was wrong. If the action they took was "right," the task is helping the family member understand how doing something "right" can result in a bad outcome because of the decisions their loved one made and the influence of the rest of the world. If the action the family member took was "wrong," the task is to help them make amends for the "wrong" and understand how a "wrong" action does not dictate a bad outcome because of the impact the loved one's ability to choose and the influence of the world have on final outcomes.

Wrong and right are in quotation marks above because their definition here is based on three criteria for guilt/shame caused by bad outcomes. Was the action taken by the family member inherently wrong? Was it in line with recovery principles? What was the motivation behind the action? Guilt from doing something inherently wrong is justified-guilt whether the outcome is good (e.g., lying keeps a friend out of jail) or bad (e.g., stealing leads to arrest). A good outcome may ameliorate guilt but usually does not erase the guilt. The way forward for inherent guilt is straightforward—making amends and forgiving.

Sebastian helping his sons use illegal substances is a good example of an intrinsic wrong. Sebastian's way forward was admitting he was wrong and making amends to himself, his sons, and his support group. An essential part of Sebastian's ability to forgive himself was understanding that helping his sons' substance use was wrong, and he was entirely responsible for helping them use. Just as important was Sebastian's understanding that his actions alone were not responsible for his sons' addiction.

The second criterion for wrongness/rightness is whether the family member's action aligned with recovery principles. If the action was in line with recovery principles, then the action was "right" whether the outcome was good or bad. An excellent example of this is a father enforcing a good boundary by refusing to let his adult child drive the family car because the son was still using substances. Shortly after the father's refusal, the son hung himself. Eric helped the father work through the guilt by telling the father that refusing to allow a person in active addiction to drive a car was the right thing to do. The loved one's response and the worldly pressures on the son led to suicide. These were beyond the father's control. If the father had let his son drive high, he could have gotten into an accident and hurt others in addition to himself. Helping the father see the "rightness" of his action ameliorated the guilt and allowed the father to grieve the loss of his son.

Conversely, if the family member's action did not align with recovery principles, as was the case for Meg, then the action was "wrong," and the recovery coach/counselor can help the family member focus their guilt on what they were responsible for—their actions and not the final outcomes. Second, help the family member make amends, give the forgiveness, and make the changes needed to align their actions with recovery principles.

The third criterion, motivation, is not usually a component in determining whether an action is right or wrong. We judge the rightness or wrongness of an action by the action itself and not what motivated a person to take that action. However, motivation is essential when identifying and mitigating guilt/shame. A noble motivation can ease the guilt/shame of a wrong action. For example, you are stealing to feed your family. Stealing is inherently wrong, but feeding your family is a noble good. Similarly, an ignoble motivation can create guilt even if the action was inherently correct and in line with recovery. For example, enforcing a boundary out of a sense of hatred and revenge can create guilt/shame even though the action was in line with good recovery practices. This guilt/shame may remain even if the outcome of enforcing a boundary is good—the loved one sought help. A good outcome may ease motivation-inspired guilt/shame but not eliminate it.

The Loved One Responds

When discussing the answers to the worksheet questions, including the loved one's role in determining outcomes is important. A family member's actions enable outcomes but do not determine them. The loved one has free will and can choose whether to respond to the family member's action constructively or destructively. The story of the Smiths and the Joneses exemplifies how a loved one's choices affect outcomes. Two different families (Smith and Jones) decided to send their loved ones to inpatient treatment. Neither of the loved ones wanted to go. Both sons resisted treatment initially but went eventually.

The Smith's son chose to run away from the inpatient facility, and eventually, the police arrested him. As of the writing of this book, Smith's son was still in active addiction. The Jones' son chose to stay and decided to embrace recovery. As of the writing of this book, the Jones' son is still in recovery. Both families made the same recovery-based decision. Their son's choices significantly impacted the outcome.

The World Responds

"The World Responds" is a catch-all category that is beyond the control of the family or the loved one. This includes genetics, environmental factors, and what other people do that impact outcomes. The key is that the family member cannot control these. Here are some ways the world can influence guilt in a family member, whether the result of the act is good or bad.

- **EXTENDED FAMILY MEMBER'S CRITICISM.** Extended family criticizes the family member for "forcing" the loved one into treatment that the loved one does not need. Similarly, if the loved one chooses to leave the home, the extended family may accuse the family member of abandoning the loved one.

- **LOVED ONE'S CRITICISM.** The loved one criticizes treatment and accuses the family member of not wanting the loved one or not caring for the loved one. This is usual, especially during the early days of treatment.

- **LOVED ONE BEGGING TO COME HOME.** This is also common in the first couple of weeks of inpatient treatment. In addition, the loved one will often promise to do whatever the family member wants and promise to remain sober.

    It is important to remember that the loved one may not be lying. The loved one may be truthful and intend to remain sober; however, they are not trustworthy in this regard because they do not have the tools they need to stay sober. It is like someone telling you they will be ten years younger tomorrow. If they believe they will be younger tomorrow, they are not lying. They are wrong. They cannot become younger. The correct response to the person in this case is, "I do not believe you can be 17 years younger tomorrow." The less accurate response is,

"I do not believe you." In the former statement, the act is being disagreed with. In the latter, you are questioning the person's integrity.

- **EXTENDED FAMILY MEMBERS OR OTHERS ENABLING THE LOVED ONE.** In one instance, the parents enforced a boundary that required the loved one to be 30 days sober to drive the family car. The loved one's grandmother allowed the loved one to use her car. The loved one wrecked the vehicle. In another instance, the aunt and uncle decided to override the parents, give the loved one a fresh start, and pay off his debts. The loved one had a major relapse. In both cases, actions beyond the control of the family member or the loved one significantly influenced the outcome of the family member's initial actions.

Parting Thoughts on Guilt and Shame

Working the 12 Steps usually brings guilt or shame issues to light and often resolves them. This worksheet is helpful if the family member is not yet working the 12 Steps, has not completed them, or has completed them, but the guilt or shame issues remain. These issues can remain after step-work completion either because God has not yet taken them away or the person's step-work did not wholly address their shame and guilt.

The benefits of holding on to guilt and shame can be a barrier to getting rid of these issues. First, focusing on the events generating the guilt/shame obviates the need to examine the family member's role in the family's dysfunction. Guilt and shame provide a place for a family member to emotionally retreat under the pretense of punishing themselves for their wrongdoing. Second, guilt/shame can give an excuse to enable a loved one or not enforce a tough boundary. Carol knew it was wrong to bail Jason out of jail. When confronted by her peer recovery coach, Carol said, "I neglected him as a child, and now I need to make it up to him." Third, after a while, the guilt and shame can become "comfortable." Guilt and shame are not pleasant, but they are familiar. There is an unquestionable comfort in the familiar.

Guilt/shame mitigation initially should focus on the event itself. Did the family member do something wrong or hurtful enough to warrant the guilt/shame they are feeling? For Eric and Carol, the answer was "No." Their children's drug use is what generated the powerful guilt/shame Eric and Carol felt, not Eric's saying "No" or Carol's not changing Jason's diaper. When looking back, Eric knew he had to be the cause of his daughter's drug use, and he was looking for the "thing" he did to cause it. Eric felt guilty because of his motive for saying no, and as Eric said, "As soon as the guilt brought the event to mind, I fixated on it as the cause of my daughter's drug use."

Sebastian's story is different. His motivation was good. He wanted to make sure his sons used substances safely. Sebastian's actions enabled his sons' out of control drug use, but they did not cause it. As illustrated in *Figure 16* above, Sebastian's "coaching" was not the sole cause of Joe's out of control drug use. Joe had to decide to take Sebastian's advice. Joe had to decide to keep using substances. Joe had to choose not to seek help when he was in the addiction (enslaved) stage of drug use. Then, the world responded to Joe's decision to use substances. In this case, Joe's environment and genetics were such that Joe transitioned rapidly to addiction (enslavement). Sebastian's "coaching" may have enabled a good outcome—Joe did not die from a drug overdose during his period of using heavily.

Helping the family members assess the true impact of their actions is a discussion of the event's immediate and long-term effects. The immediate impact of James saying "no" to his daughter was that she learned to deal with disappointment. The immediate impact on James was a sense of guilt because he believed he was being selfish.

The immediate impact of Sebastian's "coaching" is both enabling Joe's drug use and preventing an overdose. For Carol, the immediate effect on the baby was sleeping with a dirty diaper. The immediate impact for the mom was both a sense of guilt, but also she got the rest she needed. Carol was rested when she changed Jason's diaper the next day and was not as angry as she might have been if she had been tired.

The coach should assess the event's true impact on the totality of the relationship. Carol worked hard to take care of all her children. In some cases, real neglect or abuse occurs where both the immediate and long-term impacts are significant. James did a lot to support his daughter and had a good relationship with his daughter.

A client's difficulty in setting boundaries for their child is an excellent example of the latter. This client completed her step-work and worked with a recovery coach to set boundaries. Her child broke a boundary, but she was unable to enforce it because of the belief that she was a lousy parent and needed to "make it up" to the child. Despite addressing this issue in her step-work and with her coach, the problem still affected her ability to enforce boundaries. This is not uncommon. The old saying comes to mind, "Sometimes quickly, sometimes slowly."

Guilt and shame are both feelings generated by an event. Going through the EEBFA process in Chapter 14 may identify non-recovery beliefs contributing to the family member's guilt and shame. In most cases, it is the belief that an action on their part caused harm to their loved one.

CHAPTER 16

Recognizing and Dealing with Grief

Grief is an often overlooked part of SUD and codependency. Merriam-Webster defines grief as a "...deep sadness especially for the loss of someone or something loved" (Merriam-Webster 2023). Naturally, grieving is associated with the death of a loved one due to SUD, but there are other less apparent losses that the family and the loved one need to grieve. Understanding the need to grieve these less obvious losses facilitates the recovery process of the family and loved ones. The purpose of this chapter is to discuss both the loved one's grief and the family member's grief so that you will be able to:

- Explain to the family member the loved one's grief both while the loved one is using substances and when the loved one is in recovery in a manner that engenders understanding.

- Identify when a family member is grieving and bring the family member to an awareness that they are grieving.

- Provide approaches to alleviate a family member's grief.

Stages of Grief

> ### GRIEF
>
> "My daughter was an A/B student in middle school and was really good at softball and dance. I pictured her going to college, getting married and having a wonderful life. Drug addiction took hold in high school and her grades dropped and so did most of her activities. At one year into my recovery, I realized that she was an addict that I could not fix. The sadness that I felt was deep, very dark, and profound. I could almost feel the darkness gathering around me.
>
> "My productive grieving started when my counselor made me aware that I was grieving and that it was okay to grieve this loss because it was a real loss. I was journaling to begin with, but my journaling shifted to the grief that I felt. I started sharing my grief with my sponsor, my spouse, and my group. Music was one of the many coping mechanisms that recovery gave me. I learned how to play the harmonica for a comedic male beauty pageant. The harmonica became the way that I expressed the sadness I felt and helped me move past the sadness into recovery."
>
> — FAMILY GROUP MEMBER

Elisabeth Kubler-Ross (Kubler-Ross 1993) introduced the five-stage grief model in her book "On Death and Dying." The model is based on her work with terminally ill patients. Please note that there is no right or wrong way of grieving, and these stages are not meant to be linear. There is also no set time that it should take to grieve. Everyone's grief experience is different.

STAGE 1. DENIAL: The sudden change caused by the event can overwhelm an individual. This stage feels like a state of shock as the loss has not fully set in. It is a protective factor for what is to come with the other stages.

STAGE 2. ANGER: Once the truth of the loss starts to set in, an individual might experience anger. The person might express anger toward family members, toward oneself, toward God, and/or toward the addiction itself. "Why me?" is a typical thought in this stage.

STAGE 3. BARGAINING: To avoid grieving, individuals start thinking of ways to bargain. This is when the guilt is also the strongest. The use of "should of, could of, would of" is quite common at this stage. Bargaining with God is typical: "I will do this if you just do this."

STAGE 4. DEPRESSION: This is when the reality of the loss has indeed set in, and the feelings of emptiness can be overwhelming. In the depression stage, an individual might not want to be around others and could feel very foggy-headed. It is critical to move through this stage; otherwise, it can lead to being stuck in a cycle of anger and depression.

STAGE 5. ACCEPTANCE: The acceptance stage is the goal of the grieving process. When the grieving person can accept loss, they can adjust their life to include the loss and move forward with the new normal. Emotions might start to feel less like a roller coaster at this point, and previous life activities may resume.

Family Member Grief

Often, family members do not recognize they are grieving because most associate grief with the actual loss of a child or family member. Helping a family member realize they are suffering the significant losses brought about by SUD brings a great deal of relief. Some of the losses from SUD are easy to identify, like a loved one dying from SUD. Some, like those family member losses brought on by the loved one's recovery, are less obvious. A family member identifying grief when it occurs is important for two reasons. First, it brings relief to the family member. Second, the family member knows the real issue and can develop a plan to address it. One anonymous family group member shared this experience in a meeting:

> I was mad, angry, and depressed all the time. It was because of what my daughter and my wife were doing. Earlier in this meeting, Joe [fictitious name] said he was grieving the loss of his dreams for his son. It took a while for that to sink in. I just realized I am grieving the loss of the beautiful dreams I had for my daughter.

Two more takeaways from Dad's story above. First, the anger and depression were in large part due to the soul-wrenching grief caused by the loss of the dad's dreams. Second, when the dad was not aware of his grief, he blamed his intense feelings on his spouse and son. His solutions were all focused on his son and his spouse and not the grieving that was at the root of his intense feelings.

Table 4 on the next page below has other examples of the losses family members feel when their loved one is using and, surprisingly, when their loved one first becomes sober. "Dreams for a Loved One" is highlighted in both because this is quite common and particularly important to address for a family member's recovery. The dad's story above illustrates the importance of this loss. Most of the remaining losses when the loved one is using, are apparent. Loss of financial security comes from two sources. The first are the expenses associated with SUD recovery—therapy, medical fees, inpatient treatment, legal fees, and repairing damage to the home and automobile. The loved one's behavior can put the family in legal and financial jeopardy. In one instance, a family's loved one had an auto accident while using the parent's car. The accident victims sued the parents for negligence because the loved one's parents knew their loved one was using when they allowed the loved one to drive their car.

The second is the impact of SUD in the family on the wage-earner's ability to function at work or even maintain employment. Family members need to grieve emotional, mental, and physical health, relationship (including marriage) losses, and all impact one's ability to function effectively at work. Often, one spouse will quit working to take care of the loved one and address all the issues generated by the loved one's SUD.

TABLE 4. FAMILY MEMBER LOSSES WHEN THE
LOVED ONE IS USING IS IN RECOVERY

Family Member Losses When the Loved One Is Using		*Family Member Losses When the Loved One Is in Recovery*	
Financial Security	Hope	Relationship	Dreams for Loved One
Emotional Security	Marriage	Time with Loved One	Return of Sanity
Self-worth	Relationships	Routine	Comfort of Unhappiness
Self-esteem	Belief in a Higher Power	Caretaking	
Sanity	Dreams for Loved One	Sense of Purpose	
Health		Being Other-focused	

Unexpectedly, the loved one entering recovery also generates losses that the family member needs to identify and address. It is not unusual for family members to state that their lives got worse when their loved one was in recovery. Joanne said, "I thought my life would be perfect when my daughter was sober. It was not. My life got worse when she was in recovery."

As with losses while the loved one is using, some of the losses when the loved one is in recovery are obvious, and some are not. Sobriety changes the family members' relationships with their loved ones and with themselves. Sobriety changes the family's routines. The loved one may not need to be woken up for school and may find his own ride to work. These changes reduce the time the family member spends worrying about the loved one and reduce the need for caretaking.

The losses when the loved one is in recovery are important for the family member. The family members, especially parents/guardians, may lose their sense of purpose. As the loved one's SUD progresses, the loved one's sobriety becomes the focus of more of the family member's life. When the loved one becomes sober, this can leave a void because the family member no longer needs to focus on the loved one. This is especially true if the family member is not in recovery. The grief over the loss of dreams can remain with a family member for prolonged periods. In one case, the loved one was over 20 years sober and doing well. Despite the loved one's long-term sobriety, the parents still periodically grieved what their loved one lost because of addiction.

Viewing the return of sanity to the family as a loss seems odd. It is not strange when you recognize that the actual loss is the loss of excitement often associated with SUD. A wife of a recovering alcoholic said she was grateful for her husband's sobriety, but she missed the "exciting" aspects of his alcoholism. For example, the husband asked if she wanted to go to a French restaurant one evening. She said yes. He drove her to the airport. They flew to France, had dinner the next day, and flew back the following day. Eric and Joanne, driving around in the middle of the night and looking for their loved one was terrifying and exciting. Missing the "excitement" of a deadly disease may seem odd, but it does occur.

The "comfort of unhappiness" seems contradictory, but types of unhappiness can generate a certain level of comfort. First, it garners sympathy and praise. One family member talked about the adrenalin rush of having someone say, "I do not know how you are keeping it together with all that is going on in your life." Second, there is a certain level of comfort in being unhappy—less is expected of you; less is asked of you; people give you unearned breaks. In other words, it allows one to be very selfish and self-centered.

Third, it is the comfort of having only one focus—the family member's loved one. The family member's loved one has a deadly disease, so they must focus all their physical and emotional energy on the loved one. This singular focus provides family members with a ready, and some would say a commendable reason to ignore their needs, ignore other complex issues they need to deal with, and ignore other family members. The family members are unhappy with their lives, but the reason for their unhappiness allows them to ignore all the other issues in their lives. When the loved one becomes sober, other problems emerge and can overwhelm a family member.

Loved One's Grief

The substance user faces losses when they are using and, similarly, will face losses when they are in recovery. The family member needs to understand these losses so they can give their loved ones the room they need to grieve these losses. *Table 5* below lists some of the losses the loved one faces when they are using mind-altering substances and when they are in recovery.

TABLE 5. LOSSES FOR THE SUBSTANCE USER
WHEN USING AND WHEN IN RECOVERY

Losses Due to Substance Use		*Losses Due to Being in Recovery*	
Financial Security	Trust	Friends	Identity
Emotional Security	Hope	Freedom	Control
Friends	Self-Esteem	Relationship with Substance	Irresponsibility
Family	Self-Respect	Instant Gratification	Social Activities
Freedom	Sanity	Drug-induced Sense of Comfort	
Possessions	Health	Lifestyle	

The losses due to substance use are not surprising and are familiar to most family members. The losses during substance use provide the pain that can lead to the loved one seeking recovery.

Often, the family member does not understand the losses the loved one feels when they are in recovery. These losses contribute to a desire to return to using substances. One of the more surprising losses that the loved one needs to grieve is the loss of the relationship the loved one had with the mind-altering chemicals they were using. The loss of this relationship is significant and is often addressed by asking the loved one to write a farewell letter to their drug of choice.

Freedom is also in both sections. During the latter stages of substance use, the loved one loses the ability not to use and finally becomes enslaved by substance use. In recovery, a different type of freedom is lost. In recovery, the loved one loses the ability to party, go to bars, or drink with their friends. They need to say "No" to using; "No" to hanging out with old friends. They can no longer blame the substances for their wild and crazy behavior. The reality of this loss often comes out in discussions about the "wild and crazy" things they did during their drug use. This is commonly called romanticizing drug use.

One of the most challenging losses to overcome, especially for teen substance users, is the loss of the friends they used to be with. When they started using it was a ready-made group of friends- other users. Also, they could ease the grief of losing their non-using friends through their drug use.

In recovery, going back to their non-using friends is often problematic because of the bridges their drug use burned. This is why the APG is so important, especially for teens. The APG provides the opportunity to make friends who are interested in recovery.

What Can Help

Families, especially parents/guardians, often do not recognize that they are grieving. There are many things a person can try to help them through the process. Below is a list of suggested activities that might benefit anyone grieving.

- **AWARENESS.** The first step is to make them aware that they are grieving. Many times, family members do not know what is going on and will attribute what they are feeling to their loved one's drug use. Knowing they are grieving allows them to take the steps that will help them through it.

- **WRITING.** Many forms of writing can help get out the emotions of grief. Simply journaling about what an individual is experiencing, or even a guided journal, can be beneficial. Writing letters to and from God about their grief is especially helpful for a family member.

- **TALKING TO SOMEONE.** Having a trusted friend, family member, or a counselor to talk to can help to process the overwhelming feelings associated with grief. If suicidal thoughts accompany the depression stage, counseling is always encouraged.

- **PRAYER AND MEDITATION.** Meditation might be difficult, especially if there is a mental fog, but reading daily meditation books can help to calm the mind.

- **PLAYING OR LISTENING TO MUSIC.** Music is a beautiful way to express feelings of grief. Whether playing an instrument or listening to a song relatable to grief, music is healing. It reaches parts of the brain that no other method can.

- **LIVING IN THE MOMENT.** Using the living in the moment tool discussed in Chapter 12, can help family members enjoy those moments when the grief is absent. It also lets family members know that it is okay and encourages them to enjoy those good moments when they occur.

Parting Thoughts on Grief

As stated before, everyone is different and will go through the process differently. There is no right or wrong way of grieving and no time constraints on grief. Everyone is equipped with something special that can help them through these tough times, and hopefully, this is an excellent start to finding out what that is. There is light at the end of the tunnel.

Dealing with severe grief, such as the loss of a loved one, often requires specialized expertise and experience that is beyond the training of a peer recovery coach. It is essential to have resources available for the family member suffering from severe grief. Places of worship and other charitable organizations can provide no-cost or low-cost grief counseling. In some areas, there are special support groups for families who have lost someone due to addiction.

APPENDIX A

Recovery Plan Preparation

The first step is identifying the life you want by reviewing the good times when you felt most at ease and joy-filled. The second step in developing a recovery plan is identifying the assets that will assist the recovery process. Recovery assets are divided into personal assets (e.g., your strengths, talents, and gifts) and outside assets (e.g., family, church, support groups).

1. Write down at least four memories of the good times in your life in enough detail that someone else will understand them. This can be as simple as eating your favorite food as a kid, an unexpected day off from school, or as complex as a family vacation, graduating, getting an award, or getting married.

    Example: I loved having bologna sandwiches as a kid. We were poor; most of the time, it was peanut butter and jelly or egg salad. It was a special lunch when I had bologna.

2. Take a moment to read over each of these and relive them. Write down any good, positive thoughts that come to mind.

3. Look back over your life as a child, teenager, young adult, or adult and identify five or more times when you felt at ease, calm, content, or joyful. Describe them in enough detail that someone else will understand the moment.

4. Take a moment to read over each of these and relive them. Write down any good, positive thoughts that come to mind.

5. List at least four accomplishments of which you are proud.

6. Circle the activities in the table below that interest you, or you enjoy doing. Use the blanks to add others.

Go to meetings	Go to a movie	Go dancing
Talk to your sponsor	Go swimming	Listen to music
Read recovery literature	Go to the gym	Play music
Go for a walk	Go hiking	Arts and crafts
Go for a run	Photography	Work on your car
Meet with a good friend	Paint	Garden
Go to dinner	Scrapbook	Go to the beach
Have a nice meal	Hunting	Canoeing
Kayaking	Sky diving	Go to a sporting event
Watch an event on TV with friends	Go to a museum	

7. Look at the table below and circle the things at which you are good. Use the blank spaces to add anything that is missing.

Writing	Yoga	Golf
Singing	Exercise	Strategic thinking
Dancing	Weightlifting	Prophesy
Acting	Volleyball	Planning
Playing an instrument	Soccer	Counseling
Painting	Baseball	Mathematics
Sculpting	Softball	Puzzles
Football	Swimming	Strategic planning
Computer skills	Gaming	Sales
Business development	Marketing	Plan execution
Sciences	Experimentation	Exploring
Human resources	Accounting	Leading people
Plumbing	Carpentry	Electrical
Roofing	Farming	Gardening
Fishing	Auto mechanic	HVAC
Landscaping	Scuba diving	Handy person
Shooting	Archery	Flying
Construction	Plumbing	Connecting with people
Listening	Cooking/Baking	Sewing
Knitting	Crocheting	Darts
Cards	Billiards	Tennis
Other sports		

8. Review the table below and circle any outside organizations you belong to. Use the blanks to add organizations not on the list.

Church, Synagogue, Mosque, Temple	Boy Scouts	Community organizations
Fraternal Orgs (Kiwanis, Lions, Club, Masons etc.)	Girl Scouts	Volunteer organizations (Red Cross, homeless shelters, etc.)
Professional Societies	Clubs for hobbies (e.g., chess, sailing, shooting, etc.)	Other recovery support groups
Al-Anon, NAR-Anon	Mentoring (Big Brother/Big Sister etc.)	Sports clubs (football, volleyball, baseball, softball, tennis, rugby, etc.)
AA, NA, CA	School PTA	

9. What are the good things you have in your life? Circle those in the table below and add any that are not on the list in the spaces provided.

Home	Transportation	Clothing
Food	Heating/cooling	Adequate income
Health insurance	Dental insurance	Good job
Hobbies I enjoy	Good spiritual life	Good friends
Family I love	Supportive extended family	Good support groups
Good recovery program	Family and friends accept me	I am healthy
My family is healthy.	I feel loved and appreciated.	

10. An essential part of recovery is being with "winners." Winners are people who will encourage you and encourage your recovery.

   a. What traits do you think a winner for you should have?
   b. Who are the winners in your life right now, and why are they winners for you?

APPENDIX B

Codependency Recovery Plan

The purpose of this worksheet is to aid in identifying the areas that you want to include in your recovery plan.

1. Is there anything you need to work on right now?

2. Look at *Table 1* below and rate your agreement with the statement from 1 to 7, where 7 is strongly agree, 6 is agree, 5 is slightly agree, 4 is neither agree nor disagree, 3 is slightly disagree, 2 is disagree, and 1 is strongly disagree. Use the empty spaces to add any of your needs that are not covered in the table.

TABLE 1. NEEDS ASSESSMENT

Area	Statement	Level of Agreement (1-7)	Work On Now (Y/N)[21]
Body	My diet is healthy and promotes my well-being.		
	My weight is where I think it should be.		
	I am following my doctor's recommendations.		
	I am addressing medical, dental, and mental health needs.		
	I am exercising like I need to exercise.		
	I am satisfied with my physical and mental health.		
	I am not abusing mind-altering substances.		
	I have food and adequate shelter.		
	I have access to health and dental care.		
	I have an excellent job.		
	I have adequate transportation.		
	My income is sufficient to meet my needs.		
	I feel safe in my home.		

---

21 Do this after you have completed the Level of Agreement column.

Area	Statement	Level of Agreement (1-7)	Work On Now (Y/N)[21]
Mind	I know what to do when my loved one is relapsing.		
	I know what to do when I am relapsing.		
	I know all I can control is what I say, what I do, what I think, what I believe, and how I feel.		
	My beliefs are recovery beliefs.		
	I have the knowledge and tools to control what I have the power to control.		
	I know what to do when there is a crisis.		
	I understand SUD and codependency.		
	My life has a meaningful purpose.		
	I have meaningful goals.		
	I have a good understanding of each of the 12 Steps of AA.		
	I can be calm when others are in crisis.		

Area	Statement	Level of Agreement (1-7)	Work On Now (Y/N)[21]
Spirit	I have a good schedule for prayer and meditation.		
	I am hopeful for the future.		
	I routinely seek God's will for me and the courage to carry it out.		
	I have a supportive, rewarding spiritual community outside of recovery.		
	I have an intimate relationship with my Higher Power.		
	The Serenity Prayer routinely works in my life.		
	My family and friends support me in my recovery.		
	I have close, gratifying relationships.		
	My acceptance, respect, friendship, and love needs are being met.		

Area	Statement	Level of Agreement (1-7)	Work On Now (Y/N)[21]
Recovery Practices	I am going to at least one recovery meeting for myself.		
	I have supportive relationships that meet my recovery needs.		
	I am working with my sponsor and making progress in the steps.		
	I have good boundaries that I enforce with love.		
	I have replaced my unhealthy defense mechanisms with healthy recovery practices.		
	I routinely have fun with people I enjoy.		
	I have routine appointments with my recovery coach, therapist, or psychiatrist.		
	I have service/volunteer work that I enjoy.		

3. Review the statements you disagreed with in the table above—those that you rated 1, 2, 3, or 4—and select no more than three that you would like to work on now. If there are statements you agreed with—those that you rated 5, 6, or 7—that you would like to work on, annotate those statements and discuss them with your recovery coach.

4. For each statement selected, use *Table 2* on the next page to develop a plan to fill the gap in your life. *Table 3* on page 299 is an example.

TABLE 2. ACTION PLAN TEMPLATE

Goal: What do you want to accomplish?

Roadblocks	*Strengths*

Objectives: Small, concrete, time-limited steps to reach your goal

Action Step	Due Date

Person (s) to Hold You Accountable:

Appendix B: Codependency Recovery Plan

TABLE 3. EXAMPLE ACTION PLAN

Goal: What do you want to accomplish?

I want to get into shape.

Roadblocks	Strengths
I cannot afford a gym membership.	I have access to medical and dental care.
Some days, my depression is so bad that I overeat and do not feel like working out.	Other than my shoulders and depression, I am relatively healthy.
Hurt shoulders prevent me from exercising.	I have a sponsor and go to meetings.
I am afraid to start a program that I will only quit after a few weeks. This has been my pattern.	

Objectives: Small, concrete, time-limited steps to reach your goal

Action Step	Due Date
1. Make a medical appointment to have my shoulders examined.	1-May
2. Make an appointment with a therapist about my feelings of depression.	1-May
3. Research to determine if my health insurance covers gym memberships. If not, find workouts that I can do in my home.	10-May
4. Start working with my sponsor and recovery coach to overcome my fear of failure.	14-May

Person(s) to Hold You Accountable: My sponsor and recovery coach.

5. Go over each of your action plans with your recovery coach.

APPENDIX C

Plan for Enjoyment and Fun

Enjoyment and fun are essential components of recovering from codependency. It is not unusual to be so caught up in the turmoil associated with SUD, so concerned about your loved one that you forget to do the things you enjoy. Doing things you enjoy by yourself, with your family, and with friends is essential to recovery because it builds the emotional reserves needed when things are trying. The goal of this worksheet is to assist you in developing plans to have fun by yourself, with your significant other, and with your family and friends.

ENJOYMENT AND FUN BY YOURSELF

1. Take a moment and write down at least three times that you had fun or enjoyed doing something on your own. Write about each with enough specificity that you are almost reliving the event. What was the event? What did you do? What made it so memorable? How did you feel doing it? What did the air smell like? What was the weather like? What taste comes to mind when you think about it? What color? What sound?

2. Circle the activities in the table below that interest you or make you happy when you do them alone. Use the blanks to add others.

Go to meetings	Go to a movie	Go dancing
Talk to your Sponsor	Go swimming	Listen to music
Read	Go to the gym/exercise	Play Music
Go for a walk	Go hiking	Arts and crafts
Go for a run	Photography	Work on your car
Go to a museum	Paint	Gardening
Go to dinner	Scrapbooking	Go to the beach
Have a nice meal	Hunting	Canoeing
Kayaking	Sky diving	Go to a sporting event
Watch an event on TV with friends	Go fishing	Camping
Take a trip	Social media	Play computer games
Go to a park	Going to a shooting range	

3. Reexamine the activities you circled and identify those that sometimes make you feel worse when you are done. For example, social media often degrades your mood and saps rather than restores your vitality. The same can be true for some computer games.

4. Reexamine the activities you circled, find those you enjoy, and leave you feeling refreshed when you finish them.

5. Pick three things at most that you would like to do alone soon, preferably from the list of activities that leave you refreshed when you are done. Write them in the blanks below and set the date you will do it.

a. _____

b. _____

c. _____

ENJOYMENT AND FUN WITH YOUR SIGNIFICANT OTHER

1. Take a moment and write down at least three times that you had fun or enjoyed doing something with your significant other. Write about each with enough specificity that you are almost reliving the event. What was the event? What did you do? What made it so memorable? How did you feel doing it? What did the air smell like? What was the weather like? What taste comes to mind when you think about it? What color? What sound?

2. Circle the activities in the table below that interest you or make you happy when you do them with your significant other. Use the blanks to add others.

Go to meetings	Go to a movie	Go dancing
Talk to your Sponsor	Go swimming	Listen to music
Read recovery literature	Go to the gym/exercise	Play Music
Go for a walk	Go hiking	Arts and crafts
Go for a run	Photography	Work on a car
Go to a museum	Paint	Gardening
Go to dinner	Scrapbooking	Go to the beach
Have a nice meal	Hunting	Canoeing
Kayaking	Sky diving	Go to a sporting event
Watch an event on TV	Go fishing	Camping
Take a trip	Social media	Play computer games
Go to a park	Going to a shooting range	

3. Reexamine the activities you circled and find those that sometimes make you feel worse when you are done. For example, working on a car with a significant other who does not like cars may end in an argument or resentment.

4. Reexamine the activities you circled, identify those you enjoy, and leave you feeling refreshed when you finish them.

5. Pick three things at most that you would like to do with your significant other, preferably from the list of activities that leave you refreshed when you are done. Write them in the blanks below and set the date you will do it.

a. _____

b. _____

c. _____

ENJOYMENT AND FUN WITH FAMILY AND FRIENDS

1. Take a moment and write down at least three times that you had fun or enjoyed doing something with family and friends. Write about each with enough specificity that you are almost reliving the event. What was the event? What did you do? What made it so memorable? How did you feel doing it? What did the air smell like? What was the weather like? What taste comes to mind when you think about it? What color? What sound?

2. Circle the activities in the table below that interest you or make you happy when you do them with family and friends. Use the blanks to add others.

Go to meetings	Go to a movie	Go dancing
Talk to your Sponsor	Go swimming	Listen to music
Read recovery literature	Go to the gym/exercise	Play Music
Go for a walk	Go hiking	Arts and crafts
Go for a run	Photography	Work on your car
Go to a museum	Paint	Gardening
Go to dinner	Scrapbooking	Go to the beach
Have a nice meal	Hunting	Canoeing
Kayaking	Sky diving	Go to a sporting event
Watch an event on TV with friends	Go fishing	Camping
Take a trip	Social media	Play computer games
Go to a park	Throw/attend a sober party	Setting off fireworks

3. Reexamine the activities you circled and find those that sometimes make you feel worse when you are done. For example, watching an event on TV with family might not be enjoyable if your family likes to talk while watching TV and you do not.

4. Reexamine the activities you circled, find those you enjoy, and leave you feeling refreshed when you finish them.

5. Pick three things you would like to do with family and friends soon, preferably from the list of activities that refresh you when you are done. Write them in the blanks below and set the date you will do it.

   a. _____

   b. _____

   c. _____

ENJOYMENT AND FUN PLAN

This section aims to develop a realistic plan for enjoyment and fun for the next month. Realistic means you can accomplish the plan. Taking an expensive trip is not realistic if money is tight. Going hiking with your significant other is not realistic if he/she is sick or does not like to hike.

1. Spend time praying and meditating, asking your Higher Power to guide you in your selection. This time is meant to allow you to focus on what you need, not what you want. You might want to play video games alone because you are depressed and want to isolate yourself. What you might need is to either throw or attend a party.

2. Reexamine the activities you picked in each category above and write down each of those that will meet your recovery needs (not wants) and are realistic. Then, select whether you need to do the activity this week, next week, next month, or the next three months.

Activity	This Week	Next Week	Next Month	Next 3 Months
1				
2				
3				
4				
5				
6				
7				
8				

Share the table with your sponsor, counselor, significant other, or close friend, and set reasonable dates by which each will be accomplished. The purpose of sharing is to ensure the activities are restorative for you.

APPENDIX D

Codependency Relapse Prevention and Relapse Recovery Plan

A codependent relapse initiates the overwhelming desire to rescue, punish, enable your loved one, or withdraw. Withdrawing includes withdrawing from recovery, family, friends, and sometimes work. This plan has two purposes. The first is to help you prevent a relapse from occurring by identifying the warning signs of an impending relapse. The second is to help you back into recovery when you are relapsing.

FEELINGS, BEHAVIORAL CHANGES, AND TRIGGERS THAT WARN OF IMPENDING RELAPSE

Building Up to Drugging and Drinking (BUDD'ing) is a term often used to describe a loved one's relapse because the relapse starts well before they use substances. The same is true for a codependent relapse. The purpose of this section of the worksheet is to help you identify the feelings, behavioral changes, and "triggers" that precede your codependent relapse so that you can take action to prevent it.

1. Identify when you relapsed or just had a bad day with your loved one. Describe the bad day in as much detail as you can. What happened? What did your loved one do? What did you do? What did your other family members do? Who else was involved, and what did they do?

2. Identify your feelings, physical health, and mental health before and during the relapse.

    a. Before and during the relapse, what were your feelings? How did you feel? Examples include feeling hopeful because the loved one was doing well, resentful because a spouse/significant other did not follow through on a commitment, or depressed because of work, a loved one, or other family issues.

    b. Before and during the relapse, what was your physical state? Were you hungry, angry, lonely, or tired? Were you sick? Were you in physical pain? Were you neglecting your hygiene? Were you neglecting exercise? Were you eating well? Did you stop taking your medications?

    c. Before and during the relapse, what was your mental state—exhausted, overworked, lonely, depressed, anxious/agitated, hopeful, happy, or content? Did you stop taking your medications?

3. Describe your recovery program leading up to the relapse. Were you attending recovery meetings? Were you making appointments with recovery coaches/counselors? Were you talking to friends, family, or your sponsor? Was prayer and meditation part of your day? Were you taking time for yourself?

4. What was your relationship with your Higher Power before the relapse?

5. What was the state of your significant relationships before the relapse? Significant relationships could include a spouse, significant other, family, friends, pastor/priest/spiritual advisor, or boss.

6. List any significant life events before your relapse. Examples of significant life events include a death in the family, death of a friend, divorce, homelessness, significant family discord, losing a job, starting a new job, or military deployment. Did a close friend or relative die? Were there any significant issues between you and your spouse/significant other?

7. Relapsing into codependent behaviors is often due to triggers. A trigger is a singular person, place, event, or thing that can either start the codependent relapse process or lead directly to a relapse. Use the table below to identify your triggers. Use the blank spaces to add triggers that are not listed.

Seeing your loved one's dealer	Seeing people your loved one used with	Seeing the police officer who arrested your loved one
Driving by the place your loved one used	Going by the loved one's accident site	Going by your loved one's dealer's house
Loved one relapses	Loved one arrested	Money missing
Finding drugs or paraphernalia	Loved one ran away	Loved one steals your car
Call from the school	Family member criticizing you	A loved one is angry
Bad report card	Loved one asking for money	Finding stolen property
Disrespectful language	Adult loved one asking for rent/food money	A loved one is in a car accident
Manipulation	Constant badgering in person or over the phone	A loved one is upset and crying
Being judged	Loved one not getting up for school/work	Loved one asking to be rescued
My Loved one is high	Call from police	Arguing with your significant other
Seeing your loved one's car where it is not supposed to be	Seeing the backpack your loved one used for drugs	

8. Review your answers to the questions above. Think about other relapses or "awful days" and write down those that seem too often precede a codependent relapse. List them below. Share these with your sponsor and recovery coach.

KNOWING WHEN YOU ARE RELAPSING

1. During the relapse, what was your reaction when things went wrong? Did you yell, cry, plead, try "peace-at-any-price" tactics, manipulate, rescue, lie, make excuses, give up, or withdraw from life?

2. During the relapse, what were your feelings - anger, rage, resentment, hurt, self-pity, loneliness, depression, sadness, etc.? Did you feel like the world was against you?

3. What did other people say about your behavior during the relapse?

4. How did other people react to you during the relapse? What did they say? Did they withdraw from you?

STOPPING A CODEPENDENT RELAPSE BEFORE OR DURING THE RELAPSE

It is better to prevent than to try to recover from a codependent relapse. The purpose of this part of the plan is to determine what you are going to do to avoid or recover from a codependent relapse.

1. List the actions you need to take when you realize you are BUDD'ing.

2. List the actions you want others to take when you are BUDD'ing. Specifically, identify who you want to take each action.

3. List the actions you will take when something triggers you, or you realize you are relapsing.

4. List the actions you want others to take when something triggers you, or you realize you are relapsing. Specifically, identify who you want to take each action. Make sure the people you select are "winners" for you.

APPENDIX E

Suggested Reading List

This list of references and the commentary on the references. Except as noted, Phil Sagebiel wrote the commentaries for each resource below. Phil has been a family member for over ten years. He has read extensively and shares his knowledge of books designed to help families.

About Addiction and Recovery for the Whole Family

Bennett, C. (2016). *Reclaim Your Life: You and the Alcoholic/Addict* (First Edition). Sea Hill Press, Inc.

Review: This book does a fantastic job of teaching the family all about their loved one and the role the family must play in recovery. The book has these sections: 1) Identifying and understanding the person with SUD in your life; 2) Communication and boundaries; 3) You are at the helm; 4) Relapse and recovery; 5) Essays and poems. This book is aimed more at families with adult addicts (18+). See familyrecoverysolutions.com.

Bottke, A., & Kent, C. (2019). *Setting Boundaries with Your Adult Children: Six Steps to Hope and Healing for Struggling Parents*. Harvest House Publishers.

Review: The author's six steps are an acronym: SANITY. I always carry the six steps on a card in my pocket. This classic book sure helped me gain some sanity.

Brown, R., Brown, M., & Brown, P. (2014). *Families and Addiction: How to Stop the Chaos and Restore Family Balance*. February 17, 2014.

Review: This book explains skills that families need to counter the ongoing stress substance abuse causes: how to create and maintain boundaries; how to work effectively as a team; how to find and use appropriate support; how to manage the loss of trust; how to give up control of outcomes for the addict; how to give up communication with the addict and with other family members; and how to take care of yourself.

Clark, D. (2013). *Addiction Recovery: A Family's Journey*. CreateSpace Independent Publishing Platform.

Review: This book uniquely includes engaging exercises, self-assessments, and case examples. The focus of this book is on solutions and recovery for all the parties involved.

Curry, D. D. (2011). *First Aid for Enablers* (First Edition). The Rescue Mission.

Review: This book is simple yet profound in its lessons on developing healthy boundaries with the person with an addiction in your life. Chapter 5 is classic in helping enablers and their addicts get healthy and move toward recovery.

Espich, L. (2010). *Soaring Above Co-Addiction: Helping Your Loved One Get Clean While Creating the Life of Your Dreams*. Twin Feather Publishing.

Review: This is an excellent book on caring for oneself instead of becoming entangled with one's loved one.

Herzanek, J., & Herzanek, J. (2016). *Why Don't They Just Quit?: Hope for Families Struggling With Addiction*. Changing Lives Foundation.

Review: This was the first book I read regarding what family members need to know about dealing with their addicted loved one. This classic book includes much information not found in other books. If you have questions, this book has the answers. It is pretty easy to read and highly recommended.

Jay, D. (2006). *No More Letting Go: The Spirituality of Acting Against Alcoholism and Drug Addiction*. Bantam.

Review: This fabulous book focuses on what the family can and should do. I have used more quotes from this book than any other.

Jay, D. (2021). *It Takes a Family: Creating Lasting Sobriety, Togetherness, and Happiness*. Hazelden Publishing.

Review: Debra Jay has produced an incredibly detailed one-year recovery plan involving the entire family. If you like everything spelled out in intimate detail, this book is for you. See lovefirst.net.

Jay, J., & Jay, D. (2021). *Love First: A Family's Guide to Intervention* (3rd Edition). Hazelden Publishing.

Review: The first half of this book is profoundly helpful to families in understanding what is useful and what is not in relating to your loved one. The second half describes in detail how to do a family intervention. The book is fabulous, as is the related website, lovefirst.net, which includes treatment center recommendations.

Jay, J., & Borishkin, J (2007). *At Wit's End: What You Need to Know When a Loved One Is Diagnosed with Addiction and Mental Illness*. Hazelden.

Review: This book explains all the various co-occurring disorders that may be involved in addiction. Most addicts have co-occurring disorders, so this book is most helpful.

Powers, J. Z. W. (2018). *When the Servant Becomes the Master: A Comprehensive Addiction Guide* (Second Edition). Central Recovery Press.

Review: This comprehensive and understandable book provides a good understanding of addiction.

Proulx, D. A. (2021). *Understanding and Helping an Addict*. Independently Published.

Review: This is a fascinating book by a medical doctor and addiction survivor who is now a leading expert on addiction psychology. Dr Proulx describes ways for family members and loved ones to help the person with an addiction in truly effective ways. He explains how to keep your sanity when faced with the life-shattering frustration of dealing with a loved one who is self-destructing and does not want to be helped.

Schaefer, D. (1998). *Choices and Consequences: What to Do When a Teenager Uses* Alcohol/Drugs. Hazelden Publishing.

Review: This book is a fabulous, easy-to-understand book for families, teachers, and counselors that focuses on teenagers. It describes precisely what to do in a step-by-step process, which includes boundaries and contracts.

True Stories

Curry W, & Curry C. (2006). *The Lost Years (Surviving a Mother and Daughter's Worst Nightmare)*. Jeffers Press

Review: This is my favorite book among the true story categories. The mother and daughter take turns telling their side of this fantastic story with an inspirational ending.

Daxon J. (2007). *A New Normal Now.* AuthorHouse

Eric's Review: Full disclosure—Joanne Daxon, a co-author of this book, is my wife, and the story is our family's story, both during our loved ones' addiction and in early recovery. Joanne and I have given this book to family members since it was first published in 2007. Families enjoy reading the book because our story is like so many people's stories. They also want it because when you read it, you feel like Joanne is sitting across the table from you telling our story.

Gorrell, A. W., & Volf, M. (2021). *The Gravity of Joy: A Story of Being Lost and Found.* Eerdmans.

Review: The Gravity of Joy is a masterpiece of storytelling about grief, grace, and ultimate joy. If, like me, you and your family have been impacted by addiction and the opioid crisis and by untimely deaths, this book will be a salve for your soul.

West, D. (2021). *The Change Agent: How a Former College QB Sentenced to Life in Prison Transformed His World.* Post Hill Press.

Review: Wow. I will be shocked if this book does not become a movie or TV series. A big part of the author's transformation was overcoming addiction. Damon's story is both unique and inspiring. There are life-changing concepts in this true story.

Books About the 12 Steps

Beattie, M. (1992). *Codependents' Guide to the Twelve Steps* (1st Edition). Touchstone.

Review: This book is good for codependents to use for a second or third working of the Steps.

Bill P., Todd W., & Sara S. (2005). *Drop the Rock: Removing Character Defects - Steps Six and Seven* (Second Edition). Hazelden Publishing.

Review: This book is helpful to read immediately after completing your inventory.

McQ, J. (2005). *The Steps We Took* (Later Printing Edition). August House.

Review: This book is my absolute favorite for your first working of the 12 Steps, regardless of whether you have chemical or codependency issues.

APPENDIX F

Do You Need Boundaries in Your Life?

1. Look at the list below and check off the ones that apply to you. The more you check, the more you need boundaries with your loved one.

    - You are constantly walking on eggshells.
    - You are worried that you might say or do the wrong thing and do not know what the wrong thing is.
    - You dread going home because you do not know what chaos awaits you and have no idea what to do next. You doubly dread the weekends and holidays.
    - You constantly try to appease the loved one to the point that you neglect yourself and the rest of your family.
    - You invoke a consequence, later apologize to your loved one, and rescind the consequence.
    - You are hypervigilant. You are constantly watching what your loved one does. You think about your loved one all the time.
    - You cover for a loved one (lie for him, call in sick for work for her, do his homework, bail her out of jail, make excuses to the school for absences or being tardy).
    - You go out of your way to please your loved one and avoid conflict.
    - Your loved one is constantly disrespecting you.

- Your loved one is violent in the house, breaking things, punching holes in the walls, threatening, or assaulting people.
- You routinely feel resentful toward your loved one.
- You routinely feel pushed into doing things you do not want to do, especially with your loved one.
- You feel guilty saying "no" even when "no" is the correct answer.
- You believe you are responsible for your loved one's happiness.
- There is a lot of yelling and shouting in your home.
- Your loved one gets what they want by constant badgering.
- You constantly find drugs in your house and do nothing for fear of what your loved one will do.

2. Which of the above causes the most disruption in your life?

3. Which of the above causes the most fear in your life?

4. Which of the above causes the most resentment in your life?

5. Take a minute to imagine your life. If none of the statements in QUESTION 1 above apply to you, answer the questions below.

    a. What would your life be like?
    b. What would your relationship with your loved one be like?
    c. What would your relationship with your significant other be like?
    d. What would your relationships with your immediate and extended family members be like?
    e. What would your work-life be like?
    f. What would your relationship with your Higher Power be like?

APPENDIX G

Identify the Loved One's Unacceptable Behaviors and Family Member Enabling Behaviors

Boundaries are written for three reasons. The first is to identify the loved one's unacceptable behaviors. The second is to let the loved one know what you will do in response to the behavior. The third is to help you stop enabling the loved one's substance use. This worksheet is the first step in the process—identifying the behaviors.

1. Write a list of all the things your loved one does that are unacceptable to you. This can be directly drug-related behaviors—being high, drugs in the house, dealing. These can also be indirectly drug-related—lying, stealing, violence, verbal abuse, and running away. These can also be things that may not be drug-related—not doing chores, not doing homework, truancy, staying up late, and not cleaning their room. Be as thorough as possible.

2. Identify the ones that affect you the most and cause the most chaos in the house or your life. Review these and answer the following questions either for each one or for the list as a whole.

   a. How do these behaviors affect you?
   b. How is your spouse/significant other affected?
   c. How is your family affected?

3. What have you done in response to these behaviors? Has it worked?

4. Write a list of the things you do that you believe enable your loved one's substance use. Examples include yelling, shaming, giving cash, doing their homework, etc.

   a. What does your loved one gain when you do these things?
   b. What do you gain when you do these things?

APPENDIX H

Boundary-Setting Handout

1. Review the list of your loved one's unacceptable behaviors you identified previously. Write down at least three and no more than ten that are the most unacceptable to you. Review these with your recovery coach or sponsor and establish a final list.

2. For each of the unacceptable behaviors that remain, identify what you are going to do (the consequence) each time your loved one does one of these behaviors. Write it in the form of a boundary, "If you (unacceptable behavior), I will (the consequence)." Here is an example: "If I find drugs or paraphernalia, I will throw them away the first time and reevaluate your recovery plan. The second time, I will call the police."

3. For each of the boundaries above, answer the following questions:

    a. What are you gaining by not setting a boundary?

b. What will you gain by setting and enforcing this boundary?
c. What will your loved one gain if you do not set and enforce this boundary?
d. What will your loved one gain if you set and enforce this boundary?

4. Review the list of the enabling behaviors you identified previously. Write down at least three and no more than ten that are the most unacceptable to you. Review these with your recovery coach or sponsor and establish a final list.

5. Write the boundary for each of your enabling behaviors. Here is an example: "I will not give you cash until you are in long-term recovery, more than a year sober."

6. For each of boundaries above, answer the following questions:

    a. What are you gaining by not setting this boundary?
    b. What will you gain by setting and enforcing this boundary?
    c. What will your loved one gain if you do not set and enforce this boundary?
    d. What will your loved one gain if you set and enforce this boundary?

APPENDIX I

Example Boundaries for Minors and Adults

This is a list of example boundaries. This list is a starting point for creating the boundaries that work for you and your family. As always, the guidelines for boundaries apply.

EXAMPLE BOUNDARIES FOR RESPONDING TO A LOVED ONE'S ACTIONS

1. If we believe you are high, we will _____ .
   Example consequences:
   - For a minor: Make an appointment with our counselors to reevaluate your recovery plan. The new recovery plan could include a change in our boundaries, intensive outpatient treatment, partial hospitalization, or inpatient treatment.
   - For an adult: Make an appointment with our counselors to reevaluate your recovery plan. The new recovery plan could include a change in our boundaries, intensive outpatient treatment (IOP), partial hospitalization, inpatient treatment, or you are choosing to move out of our home.

If you want to allow your loved one to return home later, including the requirements for returning home is essential. Example requirements include being sober for a certain number of days, completing IOP, completing inpatient treatment, and completing aftercare requirements.

- ▶ Not allow you to drive the car (if you own the vehicle or are paying insurance) until you are 30 (or 45 or 60) days sober. The second time is 60 (or 45) days sober.
- ▶ Take or disconnect your phone until you are sober for one week (two weeks, three weeks, or ???).
- ▶ If your loved one is an adult, you can ask them to leave your home.[22]

2. If we find drugs, drug paraphernalia, or alcohol, we will _____. Example consequences:

- ▶ Throw the drugs, drug paraphernalia, or alcohol away. Alternatively, call the police and press charges if the police arrest you.
- ▶ For a minor: Make an appointment with our counselors to reevaluate your recovery plan. The new recovery plan could include a change in our boundaries, intensive outpatient treatment, partial hospitalization, or inpatient treatment.
- ▶ For an adult: Make an appointment with our counselors to reevaluate your recovery plan. The new recovery plan could include a change in our boundaries, intensive outpatient treatment, partial hospitalization, inpatient treatment, or you are choosing to move out of the house.
- ▶ Lose car privileges until you are sober for 30 days. Second time: sober 60 days. Third time: treatment.

---

22 The family member should put this boundary in place only if the loved one's actions or lack of recovery warrants it. This boundary is usually not included in the initial boundaries for your loved one.

3. If you go out without permission, leave an event or agreed-upon location without permission, or run away, we will _____. Example consequences:
   - We will call the police and list you as a runaway.
   - Car privileges will be lost for 30 days; second time: 60 days.

4. If you skip class or skip school, we will _____. Example consequences:
   - Report your absence to campus police or the school and let them know it was unexcused.

5. If there is an illegal activity (assault, taking our car without permission, dealing drugs, etc.), we will _____. Example consequences:
   - Call the police.
   - Press charges.

6. If you steal, we will _____. Example consequences:
   - Ask you to return what you stole or repay twice the value of what you stole. If you do not, we will call the police.

7. If you are disrespectful, we will _____. Example consequences:
   - Ask you to stop; we will leave the room if you do not.
   - If it escalates to violent behavior, we will call the police.

8. If you damage our home or property, _____. Example consequences:
   - You will be responsible for repairing the damage.
   - For an adult: If you do not repair the damage or pay for the repair, you are choosing not to live in our house.

9. Specific boundaries for adult loved ones living at home.
   - To live here, you must be a full-time student or pay rent.
   - If you are a full-time student and you are failing classes, you are choosing not to live here.
   - If you are not a full-time student, you must pay $_____ monthly rent. If you do not want to or if you miss two months' rent, you are choosing not to live in this house.

EXAMPLE BOUNDARIES FOR PHONE CALLS

Often, our loved ones use texts, phone calls, and emails to manipulate and act out. This is disruptive and frequently exceedingly challenging to live with. The following are sample boundaries that parents have used.

1. If you use abusive language, yell at me, or call me names in a phone call, text, or email, I will get off the phone or not answer the text or email. If you do it again, I will block you for two days.

2. If you call, text, or email trying to manipulate me or ask me for things I have already said "no" to, I will ask you to stop. If you do not, I will block you for two days.

3. If you call or text and I do not answer, please leave a message, and I will call you back. I will block you for two days if you keep calling or texting me instead.

4. It hurts me so much to listen to the terrible things happening to you when you are unwilling to get the help you need. If this type of conversation starts, I will ask you to stop. If you do not, I will hang up and block you for two days.

5. If you talk about dying or suicide, I will call the mental health unit of the police department to get you evaluated.

6. I would love to talk to you twice a day. If you call me more than that, I will not answer.

EXAMPLE BOUNDARIES FOR FAMILY MEMBER ENABLING BEHAVIORS

1. Until you are in long-term recovery, I will not give you cash.

2. For an adult loved one: I will not support you financially. The only exception is inpatient treatment.

3. I will not lie or make up excuses for you.

4. I do not condone your use of any mind-altering chemicals. This includes alcohol and marijuana.

5. I will not use illegal substances, nor will I abuse legal substances.

APPENDIX J

Resent, Own, Appreciate, Demand (ROAD) Worksheet

ROAD PROCESS USED AS A PART OF THE INVENTORY

The ROAD process will help you work through the resentments still blocking your recovery. This worksheet walks you through each of the ROAD steps. Fill out the worksheet and discuss your answers with your sponsor or coach.

RESENTMENT. The "R" stands for resentment. In this part of the process, you clearly state why you resent the person or how they harmed you in Big Book language. It is essential to be specific and brief about the harm. Focus on the harm in question.

Start by closing your eyes and, in your mind's eye, imagine the person who hurt you and fully feel your resentments. Write down each of your resentments toward the person in the form:

Person's name, I resent you for _____.

For example, "James, I resent you because you always lie to me."

This needs to be more specific. It needs to be a specific time that you vividly remember. A better way is, "James, I still resent your lying to me about where you were going last year. You told me you were going to a friend's house to study, but you went to a party with drugs and alcohol. This made me feel angry, betrayed, and frightened." The more specific the resentment is, the better.

OWN. This is where you take ownership of your part in the event. Remember, the resentment is yours now. The person who hurt you cannot change what they did and has no ownership in your resentment. Here are examples of taking ownership of the resentment in the lying example.

- "I own that I said yes even though I had no reason to trust you."
- "I own that I said yes when I knew the answer should have been no because I wanted to be the fun parent."
- "I own that I broke a boundary when I said yes to letting you go."
- "I own that I was angry when we talked."
- "I own that I got angry and said some hurtful things that I should not have said when I found out you lied."
- "I own that I did not call my sponsor before confronting you."
- "I own that I had resentments that worsened the situation."
- "I own that I used what you did as an excuse to stay in my codependence."
- "I own that my self-centeredness was a part of what took place."
- "I own that I have used this resentment in arguments with you."
- "I own that a resentment I had not dealt with caused me to be angrier at you than I should have been."

Go over the event in your mind's eye. What was your part in the event? Then write, "I own that _____."

APPRECIATE. This is the place to express gratitude for any lesson learned, either from what occurred in the past or how you have chosen to deal with the resentment. This is also the place to express understanding if there are any mitigating circumstances; express understanding if you have done something similar in your past. Talking about similar things you have done requires more explanation and a small quantity of caution.

The purpose of remembering what you did in the past is to bring compassion into your heart and your voice. It is not to absolve the person who hurt you of what they did wrong. It is not a means to justify mitigating the consequences of your loved one's actions. Sometimes, a family member will say, "I use drugs, so how can I enforce boundaries when my loved one uses drugs." This false argument falls under the line "Two wrongs do not make a right." Disclose your past similar actions only if the disclosure helps accomplish the objective of the confrontation. Examples of an "appreciate" statement:

- "I was a teenager once, and I appreciate how you would want to go to a party with all your friends."
- "I appreciate the lesson about not having and enforcing boundaries."
- "I appreciate the validation of my judgment. I knew he was not yet trustworthy, and I was correct."
- "I appreciate that as a teenager, I, too, lied to my parents."
- "I appreciate the character defects that were identified in me."
- "I appreciate that I did this to someone else."
- "I appreciate that I have lied to him."

Go over the event in your mind's eye. What do you appreciate about the event? Then write, "I appreciate that _____."

DEMAND. The demand statement is, "I demand that you stop." The purpose of this is twofold. First, it highlights that demanding someone change what they did in the past is impossible. This clarifies that the person who hurt you does not own the resentment. The resentment is yours, and you need to do what it takes to resolve it. Second, it identifies a boundary that may need to be put in place if they are still hurting you.

ROAD PROCESS USED TO CONFRONT SOMEONE LOVINGLY

This process is designed to confront someone hurting you in the present. In this case, the statements are said to the individual to get the person to stop hurting you or stop crossing a boundary you have. For this application, the ROAD process facilitates the offender's hearing what is being said and increases the chances that the offender will stop what they are doing.

RESENTMENT/HURT. In this case, the person is hurting you in the present, so it is not resentment but the hurt someone is causing you right now. However, the process is similar. Specifically, state what they are doing and how it makes you feel. The phrase that is used for this ROAD application is,

"When _____, I felt _____." Example resentment/hurt statements:

- "When I found drugs in the house, I felt betrayed, disrespected, unsafe and angry."
- "When you punched a hole in the wall, I felt scared, worried and angry."

OWN. This is your part in making the situation worse. In general, there is usually something we did that made it worse or something that we did not do that could have made it better. Examples of the scenario above:

- "I own that I got angry and said some hurtful things I should not have said."
- "I own that I did not call my sponsor before yelling at you."
- "I own that I had resentments that made the situation worse."
- "I own that I used what you did as an excuse to stay in my codependence/addiction."
- "I own that my self-centeredness was a part of this."

APPRECIATE. This is where I express my thanks for the lesson learned or express my understanding of mitigating circumstances if there are mitigating circumstances. Here are some examples of the scenario above:

- "I appreciate that you had a grueling day today."
- "I appreciate that I lied to my parents as a teenager. Like now, there were consequences for my lying."
- "I appreciate that we had a huge argument yesterday."
- "I appreciate that relapse is a part of recovery."
- "I appreciate that you are listening to me now."
- "I appreciate how this highlighted my need to work the steps with my sponsor."
- "I appreciate that I also did this to someone else."
- "I appreciate that I have done this to you in the past."

DEMAND. In this instance, you can make a demand as a boundary. For this use, it is usually better not to say, "I demand." Here are some examples of what could be said for the scenario above and other scenarios:

- "If I find drugs in the house again, I will throw them away and call your probation officer."

- "If you do not stop yelling, I will leave the room."

- "If you continue to damage the house, I will call the police."

- For adults: "By bringing drugs into our house, you are choosing not to live here."

APPENDIX K

Living in the Moment

Anxiety, fear, and anger are common in families dealing with SUD. These feelings are often generated by fearing the future or regretting the past. Many of us have had our days, and it seems our lives have been consumed by these feelings to the point that we can think of nothing else. There are times during the day, the week, and the year when our lives are really good, but we cannot enjoy them because the past or the future consumes us.

The purpose of this worksheet is to provide a tool for living in and enjoying the precious present.

1. Take a moment and determine how you are feeling right now. Write down those feelings. Are you anxious, fearful, sad, remorseful, angry, depressed, ashamed, terrified, or grieving?

2. For each of those feelings, identify what is generating that feeling. Examples include: My loved one's drug use. My loved one ran away. My loved one is in jail. I hurt my loved one. I fear my loved one will die. I regret the things I did as a parent.

3. Read the poem on the next page. What is the story saying to you?[23]

---

23 We wanted to include the poem *I Am* by Helen Mallicoat in this appendix, but we could not determine who held the copyright for the poem. Eric Daxon wrote *Where Are You?* as a poor substitute for *I Am* to try to get Ms. Mallicoat's wonderful point across.

Where Are You? by Eric Daxon (2023)

I was worrying again.
Like last night, I knew sleep would desert me tonight.
Anxiety and depression were overtaking me and
Once more, robbing me of the sleep I so desperately needed.

God said, "Where are you, Joseph?"
I was in disbelief that God was speaking so plainly to me.
Stunned is a better word.
God asked again, "Where are you?"

I understood but did not understand.
Moreover, once again, God asked gently, "Where are you, Joseph?"
With a bit of disbelief, I responded, "Lord, I am right here!"
God replied, "You are mistaken."

I fearfully responded, "But Lord, I am here.
I am here, and, unbelievably, I am here with You."
God replied, "Joseph, You are mistaken."
In desperation, I said, "But Lord, I am here! *I am here with You!*"

God patiently, sadly replied,
"You are worried about being hungry. Are you hungry now?
"You are worried about being homeless. Are you homeless now?
"My child, you are not here.
"If you were here, you would be enjoying a full stomach and a roof over your head.
"Yet you are not.

"You are in yesterday worried about the mistakes you made in the past.
"You are in the future, worried about what might happen next.
"You are not here. If you were here, you would be with Me."
God paused. I shuddered. God continued,

"I am in 'the here' and not the 'was' nor the 'will be.' I am here.
"Rest with Me now, Joseph. Rest with Me in the 'here.'
"When tomorrow becomes 'here', I will be there too. Rest, my child."
I understood. I smiled. I slept. Oh, how I slept!

I slept knowing that when tomorrow became today,
God would be with me in tomorrow's here.

4. Carefully examine the moment you are in right now. Describe this moment. Describe what is going on around you right now. Answer the questions below to aid in this assessment.

    a. Are your physical needs—food, water, shelter, security—being met?
    b. Is there anything you need (the word is need, as in must do before the session is over) to do right now, as in this instant? If the answer is "Yes," please do them.

5. Dawn, a family member, relayed the following story about her teenage loved one:

    After one of our hardest seasons with our teen, I frequently thought about how horrible the entire year was, and it kept me feeling so heavy and so sad. But when I challenged myself to really consider how many bad days there were ... days with fighting [with her teen] or [her teen] sneaking out or getting a call from the school...there were thirty? Maybe sixty? And that left three hundred medium and even good days to focus on. That shift in perspective eventually helped me view our life and our child in a more positive light, even as our struggles continued.

    a. What is the story you tell people about your life since SUD entered your family?
    b. How does the story you tell make you feel?
    c. As Dawn did, take a moment and examine what your life has been like since SUD entered your life. Were there good times?
    d. Are these "good times" a part of the story you tell others and yourself?

6. Act as if, at this moment, you could let go of regretting the past and let go of worrying about the future. What will you gain? How would you feel? What do the good times described above tell you about your life if you choose to see the past and the present clearly?

APPENDIX L

AA Big Book Prayers, Your Higher Power Speaking to You

Our Higher Power speaks to us in many ways. One way is through prayer. Many have experienced that God will use the same recovery meditation, passage in the Bible, quote in the Big Book, or saying to tell us different things when He needs us to know them. As life circumstances change and our relationship with our Higher Power changes, He reveals another message. The purpose of this exercise is to see what your Higher Power is using the prayers in the Big Book to reveal to you today. All the prayers are taken from AA World Services, Inc. Big Book (Alcoholics Anonymous 2019).

Third Step Prayer

God, I offer myself to Thee—to build with me and to do with me as Thou wilt. Relieve me of the bondage of self, that I may better do Thy will. Take away my difficulties, that victory over them may bear witness to those I would help of Thy power, Thy love, and Thy Way of life. May I do Thy will always! AA Big Book page 33 (Alcoholics Anonymous 2019).

1. What message did this prayer give you the first time you read it? What is God trying to tell you today? If this is your first time reading the prayer, focus on the message you are receiving now. If your initial answer is that you received no message, reread the passage and wait.

2. "Bondage of self." What shackle prevents you from acting on your decision in Step 3?

Seventh Step Prayer

"My Creator, I am now willing that you should have all of me, good and bad. I pray that you now remove from me every single defect of character that stands in the way of my usefulness to you and my fellows. Grant me strength, as I go out from here, to do your bidding. Amen." AA Big Book on page 76.

1. What message did this prayer give you the first time you read it?

2. What message is this prayer giving you today?

3. Are you willing to accept who you are today, including your character strengths and defects? Do you have a choice? Please explain.

QUESTIONS RELATED TO BOTH PRAYERS

These questions relate to all the prayers above. Please review the prayers again and answer the following questions:

1. If an author repeats something, it is essential to the author. Please answer the following questions:

    a. From your perspective, what concepts repeat in each of the prayers?
    b. How successful are you in implementing these common concepts?
    c. What are your roadblocks?
    d. What will you gain by overcoming the roadblocks?

2. After re-reading all the prayers, what insights do you have about yourself? Your relationship with God? God's love for you?

3. Read and meditate on the passage below. Look at your eyes in a mirror, and what do you see? If you saw yourself as God sees you, what would you see?

"You will never look into the eyes of someone God does not love." Anonymous[24]

---

24 The author of this statement is listed as anonymous. AZQuotes.com lists Bill Hybels, but we could not verify this.

APPENDIX M

Prayer and Meditation

Prayer and meditation are an essential part of any recovery program. In the AA Eleventh Step prayer and meditation are the keys to implementing the decision to turn our will and lives over to our Higher Power. The purpose of this worksheet is to foster an improvement in your prayer and meditation.

"Every one of us needs half an hour of prayer a day, except when we are busy—then we need an hour." St. Francis de Sales

"I used to believe that prayer changes things, but now I know that prayer changes us, and we change things."[25] Saint Teresa of Calcutta

PRAYER AND MEDITATION

1. How has your prayer and meditation changed from when you started? If you are beginning, describe your prayer and meditation and how you would like it to be.

2. What are your primary roadblocks to daily prayer and meditation? How can you overcome them?

---

25   https://www.azquotes.com/quote/813569. Last accessed April 28, 2020

3. What are you getting from failing to pray and meditate daily?

4. What do you have to gain by praying and meditating daily?

5. Why, in your opinion, does St. Francis de Sales recommend more, not less, time praying (an hour vs a half hour) if you are busy?

6. What does St. Teresa of Calcutta mean when she says, "I used to believe that prayer changes things, but now I believe prayer changes us and we change things."? Do you agree?

EXAMINE YOUR PRAYER

"God speaks in the silence of the heart. Listening is the beginning of prayer."—St. Teresa of Calcutta.

1. What is the most intimate thing you have shared with God?

    Sharing with God means consciously communicating this to God in thought or direct verbalization. This can be an event, a character flaw, something you are ashamed of or feel guilty about, a significant decision you are thinking about, a deep feeling, or what you think about God.

2. Have you ever been less than honest about sharing with God? Have you ever "hidden" something from your Higher Power?

    "Less than honest" can take many forms. The first is deception. Something like, "I am grateful for all I have," when you are upset that your bank account is not big enough. The second is hiding something you did or are doing. Hiding can take a couple of forms. One form hides behind rote prayers, so you do not talk to God. Rote prayers are good and serve a good purpose for focusing the mind. However, they are often used to hurry through your time with God so that you can say you were praying.

Another form of hiding can be walling off an area you treat as separate, not a part of you. This is usually because of shame but can be because of trauma. For men, pornography is often a walled-off area. Another walled-off area can be past abuse or abuse that you have perpetrated. This can be the hardest to identify because it is something that you naturally hide and do not want to consider to be a part of you. Please answer the following questions:

a. Have you ever been dishonest in your prayers with God? Please describe.
b. Have you ever hidden behind rote prayers? Please describe.
c. Are you walling off areas in your life? If so, what are they?
d. What is blocking you from intimately sharing your life with God daily?

3. Hiding feelings from God builds a wall that will hinder the development of a more intimate relationship. What feelings have you hidden, or are you hiding from God? List them, select the one most important to you, and write it in the format below.

God, I have not shared the compulsion to drink with You. I tried to overcome this feeling on my own and often failed. I want to share this with You now. On my way home, I felt a desire for my first drink. That desire pushed You out of my thoughts. I wanted to have just one drink. After the first drink, I felt the desire for another drink. After the second drink, desire turned into shame and guilt that I did not share with You. I was convinced that I could control it next time. I am sharing the lust for a drink and the shame with You now in the hope that when they come again, I will immediately recognize the feelings for what they are, immediately share them with You, and finally, share them with someone I trust. Anonymous Family Group Member

4. Step 11 says, "...praying only for knowledge of his will for us and the power to carry that out." Is this a part of your prayer? Why is this so important?

EXAMINE YOUR MEDITATION

As in any good relationship, there is a time for talking and a time for listening. In meditation, we listen to God. This is often harder than it sounds. Forgetting ourselves and listening to God can take time and much practice because so much of our lives are spent on self-centered thought.

1. What are the purposes of meditation in a recovery program?

2. Describe how you meditate.

3. How does your Higher Power communicate with you when you meditate?

APPENDIX N

Worksheet for the Event, Emotion, Belief, Feeling, Action Process

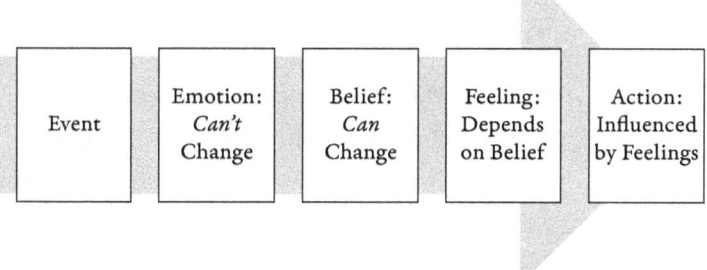

EVENT, EMOTION, BELIEF, FEELING, ACTION

The figure above shows most people's basic response process to an event. An event evokes an innate emotion. For this exercise, an emotion is the body's immediate, unthinking reaction to the event. A pre-event belief about the emotion or the event leads to a feeling. The feeling influences the action that will be taken. Here is a simple example. Your loved one relapses. This generates the emotion of fear. You believe your loved one purposely does this to you as an act of defiance. This causes feelings of being insulted, betrayed, disrespected, and angry. You yell at your loved one.

EEBFA WORKSHEET

The worksheet's purpose is first to reexamine the impact of your beliefs on you, your loved one, and your family. Second, it is to help you develop new beliefs concerning the events that led to and are currently causing chaos in your life.

1. **IDENTIFY THE EVENTS.** First, list what your loved one did that caused you and your family pain, anger, or chaos. Events could be a relapse, arrest, finding drugs, coming home high, giving drugs to a sibling, stealing, failing a class, truancy, yelling and shouting, being disrespectful, or violence.

2. **SELECT THREE OF THE MOST SIGNIFICANT EVENTS.** These could be events that caused the most harm, events that hurt you, and events that still bring up resentments when you remember them.

3. **BRIEFLY DESCRIBE ONE OF THE EVENTS.** Describe the event in enough detail so that someone else will understand how the event hurt you or your family.

4. **IDENTIFY THE EMOTION YOU FELT.** Think about the encounter and focus on when you knew something was wrong. The moment you smelled alcohol in your loved one's breath. The moment you knew they had relapsed. The moment you knew the car was missing. The moment your loved one started yelling at you. The moment you heard the police officer say they had your loved one in custody.

What was your immediate reaction or emotion? For this worksheet, use one of these six emotions: love, joy, anger, sadness, fear, or surprise.

5. **IDENTIFY THE FEELING.** How did you feel after the initial emotion subsided? The emotion of surprise at smelling alcohol might have turned into the feeling of anger. Some emotions can also be feelings. The difference is that emotion is a spontaneous response to an event you cannot control. It is a biochemical response. A feeling is longer-term.

6. **IDENTIFY THE ACTION.** What did you do (yell, call names, kick them out of the house, belittle them, punish them, etc.)?

7. **IDENTIFY THE BELIEF.** Identify the belief you had about the event. Use the lists of non-recovery beliefs and recovery beliefs below as a guide.

8. **CHANGE THE CODEPENDENT BELIEF TO A RECOVERY BELIEF.** Replace the codependent belief with a recovery belief. Replay the event with the recovery belief. How did your feelings change when you replayed the event with the recovery belief? How did your actions change?

9. Which belief system was more effective for you and your loved one?

NON-RECOVERY BELIEF SYSTEM

The codependent or uninformed belief system makes recovery more complex. Example beliefs include:

- Using is a lack of willpower. They could stop if they wanted to.
- It is my fault they are using substances. I caused this because I did not parent correctly.
- I can fix this. I can get them to stop.
- It is just a phase. I do not need to do anything. They will snap out of it.
- I can save them.
- My loved one needs help. I do not need help. I do not need a recovery program.
- I can control my loved one's behavior.
- I can guilt and shame them into doing what I want them to do.
- How can they do this to me after all I have done for them?
- I will bail them out again to get them on the right track. Then things will be okay.
- Letting go and detaching are the same as giving up.
- My loved one cannot recover without my help.
- If I love them, I should trust them.
- If I love them, I should like them.
- I can love them out of this disease. If I love them enough, they will quit.
- I am responsible for the outcomes.
- God's plan is not working, so I will take over.

RECOVERY BELIEF SYSTEM

There are core beliefs that foster recovery from codependency and addiction. Key beliefs include:

- Addiction is a disease. This is the fundamental belief that allows responding versus reacting. It also is the basis for each of the remaining beliefs. The addiction process started with a choice—the choice to use.

- Addiction affects the whole family. The entire family needs help.

- The 3 C's. You did not cause the disease, you cannot control them, and you cannot cure them.

- Recovery cannot be done alone; however, each person is responsible for their recovery. You cannot work someone else's program for them.

- Enabling a loved one's recovery means allowing them to feel the natural consequences of their substance use.

- This is a program of unconditional love, not unconditional trust nor unconditional like. Love is given. Trust and "like" are earned.

- Letting go and detaching foster recovery in you and your loved one.

- I can control only what I say, what I do, what I think, what I believe, and how I feel.

- God's plan and not my plan. My Higher Power has a plan for my loved one and me. My task is to seek God's plan for me and let my loved one do the same.

APPENDIX O

Guilt and Shame Inventory

This worksheet aims to help identify the source of guilt or shame that may block your recovery. Once the source of the guilt/shame is identified, your recovery coach can help you do the "next right thing" to resolve these lingering and often debilitating feelings.

1. List any past or current events that generate guilt or shame. The event could be something you did—I stole from my parents. The event can be something you did not do—I did not enforce a boundary. It can be something someone did to you—my dad got drunk, and I believed it was because I was not good enough.

2. Relive the event in your mind's eye, and without ascribing blame, fully describe each event you listed in QUESTION 1 as best as you can remember it. Be as factual as you can be. Include in the description the following:

    a. Accurately describe what happened. What specifically did you do? If another person was involved, what did they do?

b. If you did wrong, state precisely what you did wrong. If the other person did wrong, state what they did wrong.

c. State precisely how you harmed another person, yourself, or someone harmed you.

3. Guilt/shame are often associated with an event. Sometimes, your memory of the event you carry with you daily is inaccurate or incomplete. Sometimes, the inaccuracies or what was left out is the source of unwarranted guilt/shame. Reexamine what you have written in QUESTION 1 and QUESTION 2 and answer the following questions:

   a. Compare your day-to-day memory of the event listed in QUESTION 1 with what you wrote about it in QUESTION 2. Are they the same? If not, what are the differences?

   b. For each event, what is the next right thing for you to do today? If you hurt someone, you may need to make amends. If someone hurt you, forgiveness may be in order. If your guilt was unjustified, you did nothing wrong, letting go of the false guilt may be in order.

   c. What are the barriers, if any, stopping you from doing the next right thing?

4. Discuss your answers with your coach.

Cloud, William, and Robert Granfield. 2008. "Conceptualizing Recovery Capital: Expansion of a Theoretical Construct." *Substance Use & Misuse* 1971-1986.

Codependents Anonymous. n.d. *What is Codependence?* Accessed September 2021. https://coda.org/newcomers/what-is-codependence/.

Collier, Crystal, Robert Hilliker, and Anthony Onwuegbusie. 2014. "Alternative Peer Group: A Model for Youth Recovery." *Journal of Groups in Addiction and Recovery* 9 (1): 40-53. doi:10.1080/1556035X.2013.836899.

Copland, Mary. 2018. *Wellness Recovery Action Plan.* Sudbury, MA: Human Potential Press.

D., Joanne. 2007. *A New Normal Now.* Bloomington, IN: AuthorHouse.

Delgado, J. 2020. Accessed April 2020. https://psychology-spot.com/list-of-emotions-and-feelings/.

Drug Enforcement Agency. 2023. *Fentanyl Awareness.* https://www.dea.gov/fentanylawareness.

Hampton, Debbie. 2015. *What is the Difference between Feelings and Emotions?* January 12. Accessed 2020 April. https://thebestbrainpossible.com/whats-the-difference-between-feelings-and-emotions.

Hybels, Bill. 2020. "Bill Hybels Quotes." *AZQUOTES.* May 10. https://www.azquotes.com/author/29869-Bill_Hybels.

Jay, Debra. 2006. *No More Letting Go: The Spirituality of Taking Action Against Alcoholism and Drug Addiction.* New York, New York: Bantam Dell.

Kubler-Ross, Elisabeth. 1993. *On Death and Dying.* Chicago.

Lancer, Darlene. 2017. "Codependency Addiction: Stages of Disease and Recovery." *Global Journal of Addiction & Rehabilitation Medicine* (Juniper Publishers) 2 (2): 21-22.

Mallicoat, Helen. 2020. *"I Am" (Helen Mallicoat).* May 27. https://soulpatch.net/2013/06/21/i-am-helen-mallicoat/.

2017. *Pleasure Unwoven.* Internet Video. Directed by Kevin McCauley. Performed by Kevin McCauley. Accessed May 12, 2023. https://www.youtube.com/playlist?list=PLYCfN98iD1frkbkvTVjKr2U2KciDMMtWy.

McLellan, A. Thomas. 2017. "Substance Misuse and Substance Use Disorders: Why Do They Matter in Healthcare?" *Transactions of the American Clinical and Climatological Association* 128: 112-130.

McNeely, J., and A. Adam. 2020. *Substance Use Screening and Risk Assessment in Adults [Internet} Table 3, DSM-5 Diagnostic Criteria for Diagnosing and Classifying Substance Use Disorders.* Baltimore, MD, OCT. Accessed February 15, 2023. https://www.ncbi.nlm.nih.gov/books/NBK65474/Table/nycgsubuse.tab9/.

Meehan, Bob. 2007. *Beyond the Yellow Brick Road: Our Children and Drugs, Revised.* Roswell, GA: Meek Publishing.

References

AA Agnostica. 2023. *AA Agnostica Home.* May 22. Accessed May 22, 2023. https://aaagnostica.org/.

—. 2012. "A-Collection-of-Alternative-Steps-2012-07-09." *AA Agnostica.* July 9. Accessed May 22, 2023. https://aaagnostica.org/wp-content/uploads/2012/07/A-Collection-of-Alternative-Steps-2012-07-09.pdf.

Al-Anon Family Groups. 2011. *Many Voices, One Journey.* Virginia Beach, VA: Al-Anon Family Group Headquarters.

Alcoholics Anonymous. 2019. *Alcoholics Anonymous.* Fourth Edition. New York, New York: Alcoholics Anonymous World Services, Inc.

American Psychiatric Association. 2013. *American Psychiatric Association: Diagnostic Statistical Manual of Mental Disorders.* Fifth. Arlington, VA.

—. 2020. *What Is a Substance Use Disorder?* December. Accessed November 19, 2021. https://www.psychiatry.org/patients-families/addiction-substance-use-disorder/what-is-a-substance-use-disorder.

American Psychological Association. 2023. *APA Dictionary of Psychology.* July 14. Accessed July 14, 2023. https://dictionary.apa.org/codependency.

Beattie, Melody. 1992. *Codependent No More: How to Stop Controlling Others and Start Caring for Yourself.* 2nd. Center City, MN: Hazeldon.

Blackburn Center. 2020. *Nice vs Kind: Why Does It Matter?* July 7. Accessed September 2021. https://www.blackburncenter.org/post/nice-vs-kind-why-does-it-matter.

Caparrotta, Martin. 2020. *Being Nice vs Kind - What's the Difference? (8 Experts Explain).* November 2. Accessed September 2021. https://humanwindow.com/nice-vs-kind.

Cates, John C, and Jennifer Cummings. 2003. *Recovering Our Children: A Handbook for Parents of Young People in Early Recovery.* New York, Lincoln, Shanghai: Writers Club.

Chand, S, D Kuckel, and M Hueker. 2024. "Cognitive Behavioral Therapy." In *StatPearls.* Treasure Island, FL: StatPearls Publishing. Accessed March 10, 2024. file:///C:/Users/ericg/Zotero/storage/4TI9P4ZE/NBK470241.html.

Churchill, Winston. n.d. *Winston Churchill Quotes.* Accessed May 2020. https://www.azquotes.com/quote/404902.

Cloud, Henry, and John Townsend. 1992. *Boundaries.* Grand Rapids, MI: Zondervan.

—. 2007. *Beyond the Yellow Brick Road: Our Children and Drugs, Revised.* Roswell, GA: Meek Publishing.

Merriam-Webster. 2023. *Grief Definition & Meaning.* Accessed November 24, 2023. https://www.merriam-webster.com/dictionary/grief.

—. 2023. *Self-will.* Accessed November 22, 2023. https://www.merriam-webster.com/dictionary/self-will#:~:text=%3A%20stubborn%20or%20willful%20adherence%20to%20one's%20own%20desires%20or%20ideas%20%3A%20obstinacy.

Miller, William R, and Rollnick Stephen. 2013. *Motivational Interviewing: Helping People Change.* Third. New York: The Gilford Press.

Nash, Angela, and Chrystal Collier. 2016. "The Alternative Peer Group: A Developmentally Appropriate Support Model for Adolescents." *Journal of Addictions Nursing* 27 (2): 109-119. doi:10.1097/JAN.0000000000000122.

National Institute on Drug Abuse. 2020. *Drugs, Brains, and Behavior: The Science of Addiction Drug Misuse and Addiction.* July 13. Accessed March 2021. https://www.drugabuse.gov/publications/drugs-brains-behavior-science-addiction/drug-misuse-addiction#ref.

Nowinski, Joseph. 2011. *The Family Recovery Program.* 2nd. Hazelden.

Palmer Drug Abuse Program - National, Inc. 1982. *Fists and Hearts: The Story of PDAP.* Dallas, TX: Palmer Drug Abuse Progam - National, Inc.

Palmer Drug Abuse Program. 1990. *PDAP (Also called the PDAP White Book).* Midland, Texas: Palmer Drug Abuse Program Services Inc.

PaulChapman.com. 2019. *4 Types of Love (Agape. Phileo,..).* August 3. Accessed March 2021. https://paulechapman.com/?s=agape+love.

PDAP. 1982. *Fists & Hearts: The Story of PDAP.* Dallas, TX: PDAP National, Inc.

—. 1990. *PDAP : The White Book.* 2nd. MIdland, TX: PDAP.

Powers, Jason Z.W.,. 2012. *When the Servant Becomes the Master.* Las Vegas: Central Recovery Press.

Prochaska JO, DiClemente CC, Norcross JC. 1992. "In Search of How People Change: Applications to Addictive Behaviors." *Am Psychol*, Sep: 1002-14. Accessed Jan 2022. doi:10.1037//0003-066x.47.9.1102.

Shaefer, Dick. 1998. *Choices and Consequences: What to Do When a Teenager Uses Alcohol/Drugs.* Hazelden Foundation.

Shaver, P, J Schwartz, D Kirson, and C O'Connor. 1987. "Emotion Knowledge: Further Exploration of a Prototype Approach." *Journal of Personality and Social Psychology* 1061-86.

Shi, Kelly. 2016. *Being Nice vs Being Kind.* April 26. Accessed September 2021. https://www.scu.edu/the-big-q/being-nice-vs-being-kind/.

SMART Recovery. 2024. *Learn About SMART Recovery*. Accessed January 11, 2024. https://smartrecovery.org/what-is-smart-recovery.

Song For Charlie. 2023. *https:/www.songforcharlie.org*. March 8. Accessed March 2023.

Spencer, Maya. 2012. *Spirituality*. Accessed March 10, 2024. https://www.rcpsych.ac.uk/docs/default-source/members/sigs/spirituality-spsig/what-is-spirituality-maya-spencer-x.pdf?sfvrsn=f28df052_2.

Steps of Faith. 2020. *The Seven Types of Love in the Bible*. Feb 18. Accessed November 2021. https://steppesoffaith-56895.medium.com/the-7-types-of-love-in-the-bible.

Substance Abuse and Mental Health Administration. 2014. *SAMHSA's Concept of Trauma and Guidance for a Trauma-Informed Approach*. Office of Policy, Planning, and Innovation, SAMHSA, Rockville, MD: SAMHSA. Accessed March 10, 2024. https://store.samhsa.gov/sites/default/files/sma14-4884.pdf.

Substance Abuse and Mental Health Services Administration. 2012. "SAMHSA's Working Definition of Recovery: 10 Guiding Principles of Recovery." Edited by SAMHSA. February. Accessed March 10, 2024. https://store.samhsa.gov/product/SAMHSA-s-Working-Definition-of-Recovery/PEP12-RECDEF.

Substance Abuse and Mental Health Services Administration. 2020. *Substance Use Disorder and Family Therapy - TIP 39*. SAMHSA.

U.S. Department of Health and Human Services (HHS). 2016. *Facing Addiction in America: The Surgeon General's Report on Alcohol, Drugs, and Addiction*. Office of the Surgeon General, Washington, D.C.: HHS.

White, Mary Gormandy. n.d. *Powerful Greek Words for Love & Their Meanings*. Accessed November 2021. https://reference.yourdictionary.com/other-languages/powerful-greek-words-love-their-meanings.

White, William L., and William Cloud. 2008. "Recovery Capital: A Primer for Addiction Professionals." *Counselor* 22-27.

www.ingramcontent.com/pod-product-compliance
Lightning Source LLC
Chambersburg PA
CBHW020531030426
42337CB00013B/806